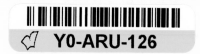

MIND/BODY FITNESS

Mind/Body Fitness

focus preparation performance

TOM SEABOURNE, PH.D.

Strategies for Success from a Champion Martial Artist

YMAA PUBLICATION CENTER
Boston, Mass. USA

Publisher's Cataloging in Publication
(Prepared by Quality Books Inc.)

Seabourne, Thomas.
    Mind/body fitness : focus, preparation, performance /
by Tom Seabourne. -- 1st ed.
    p. cm.
    Includes bibliographical references and index.
    LCCN: 00-106042
    ISBN: 1-886969-87-6

    1. Health. 2. Physical fitness. 3. Martial arts.
I. Title.

RA781.S43 2001   613.7'148
                  QBI00-790

Edited by Sharon Rose
Text and Cover Design by Katya Popova
Cover Art courtesy of Art Resource

Disclaimer:
    The authors and publisher of this material are NOT RESPONSIBLE in any manner whatsoever for any injury which may occur through reading or following the instructions in this manual.
    The activities, physical or otherwise, described in this material may be too strenuous or dangerous for some people, and the reader(s) should consult a physician before engaging in them.

Printed in Canada.
10 9 8 7 6 5 4 3 2 1

YMAA PUBLICATION CENTER
Main Office: 4354 Washington Street
Boston, Massachusetts, 02131
617-323-7215 • 1-800-669-8892
www.ymaa.com • ymaa@aol.com

*This book is dedicated to those readers, writers, teachers,
students, martial artists, and sports enthusiasts,
who commit their lives educating themselves
to make a difference. These individuals
get up every morning, find a purpose,
and wake up the world with
their philosophies.*

❋

Contents

❋ Foreword ❋

I HAD THE GREAT FORTUNE of meeting Tom Seabourne more than twenty years ago, through his martial arts and tennis classes. The techniques and philosophies about fitness and energy that Tom shared with me have improved my performance in all the sports I practice—including cycling, hiking, and yoga. Moreover, Tom's insight has helped me tremendously in the business world: preparing for stressful meetings, giving presentations, dealing with a hectic travel schedule, and meeting all of the challenges faced by an entrepreneur.

I have always admired people who function at an extremely high level—and Tom is certainly one. I have observed his ability to be completely relaxed while sparring, deliver a killer punch in a burst of energy, then return to a relaxed posture with his guard still up. He is an advocate for a good metaphor for life—relaxed awareness.

Tom is truly a master of multitasking, that revered quality that enables you to juggle myriad things at once, while successfully completing each one. He has perfected the ability to focus intently on a number of topics simultaneously, devoting the necessary time to each without slighting any one. Tom has an exceptional ability to combine the wisdom of his martial arts training and academic background in sports psychology and philosophy, and extract solid practical advice for people who seek to reduce stress while working and training more efficiently. He demonstrates that through mindfulness, it is possible to accomplish a surprising number of things in a day, and yet feel energized throughout the process.

One of the greatest benefits to a mindful mindset is the enhanced recall of events. By consciously focusing on a pleasurable moment while it's in progress—being completely aware of as many details as possible, including sounds, smells, colors, etc.—I can reconstruct the event and benefit more than once from this pleasant memory. At times this requires actually stopping and taking a deep breath—for example, during an ascent on a hike simply to admire the view. Observing the sky, trail, rocks, etc. will create a more mindful experience, and enable you to focus on more than just attaining the summit of the mountain.

Several years ago, I realized a lifelong dream and embarked on a solo world tour, with just a backpack and thick address book. My days were filled with overwhelming sights and sounds; I tried to write my observations in a journal, but I was often too exhausted. Conscious of my incredible fortune to have the time, resources, and energy to complete such a trip, the minor inconveniences dissipated. The lack of hot water, timely meals, predictable trains, etc. was insignificant compared to the rich experiences I was accumulating. I relive these precious memories almost daily: the awe of meditating alone inside one of the Great Pyramids of Egypt, or walking along the Great Wall of China at sunset. Mindful recollection of these exhilarating moments can sustain my spirit indefinitely.

The positive effects of the mind/body connection are especially critical when training, and the applications are endless. Mindfulness is essential while practicing yoga. The most satisfying sessions are those in which I do not look at the other participants, but focus solely on my breathing and the voice of the instructor, while staring at a place somewhere ahead of me. In such a mindful state, the muscles are relaxed and more malleable, and it's possible to achieve my personal best performance.

In tennis, maintaining a mindful state can be extremely helpful. For example, Tom instructed me to focus on my breathing as well as on my strokes and footwork. The face of my opponent becomes blank and irrelevant, as I visualize a strong, powerful stroke, placing the ball exactly where I want it.

The endorphin release I get from rollerblading is intense—I make sure to leave the cell phone and Walkman at the office and truly enjoy the escape. I often take morning beach walks, and the sound of the waves stays with me all day. When thoughts of a work problem or family challenge seep in, I try to banish them and refocus on the beauty of the moment at hand. Mindfulness means full awareness of your senses, even if sometimes you are required to repeatedly dispense with negative feelings. With some practice, this is possible in even the most stressful environments.

My best friend and I recently escaped for three days of hiking at Big Sur National Park. Near the trailhead, we passed a phone booth, and she felt compelled to check her voicemail. Sure enough, her obsessive/compulsive boss had phoned, leaving several frantic messages. There ensued forty minutes of phone calls, leaving my friend stressed and unable to relax and enjoy the beauty of the Pacific Ocean in front of us. I sat waiting nearby on a rock, then reiterated how I was unwilling to let her boss ruin our weekend. We laughed and took deep breaths, determined to refocus on the gorgeous scenery and fresh air. I threatened to make her walk home if she called the office again! I was determined not to let my friend's anxiety permeate our tranquil environment, and it worked—the hikes were amazing, and we enjoyed great conversations by the fire each evening.

A state of mindfulness while practicing sports can certainly enhance performance, and the same is true in the intellectual realm. Recently, I was studying for my MBA while working full-time and traveling overseas frequently. It was the most stressful two years of my life. I became a master at multitasking, which meant I could accomplish a great deal without giving my full attention to anything. Distracted by school deadlines, I made stupid mistakes at work. I vowed to remain mindful of my daily responsibilities at work, and then switch gears while listening to music during the drive to campus. I made long "To Do" lists and tackled them, focusing on the most critical tasks. My goal was to be a good team member at work and at school, while staying as healthy as possible and completing my MBA. I rewarded myself for these intense study periods with relaxing evenings with family and friends—consciously blocking out all worries regarding school or work. It wasn't easy, but it was critical to my peace of mind.

My work now involves mostly left brain, analytical thinking; sometimes involving as many as seventy-five phone calls, punctuated by as many emails, and report writing in a day. In between these activities, I relax and refocus by doing stretches on the floor (sometimes while wearing my telephone headset!). During long elevator rides on my way to meetings, I often do wall slides. People sometimes stare, but their legs don't feel as good as mine afterwards.

I frequently take ten-hour nonstop flights to Europe, and used to arrive exhausted and achy. By incorporating meditation, stretching, good nutrition, and adequate hydration, I now proceed straight to my meetings. Instead of dwelling on the stressful airport arrival as the trip progresses, I concentrate on the clouds and the pure luxury of floating in such a peaceful place. It helps to be mindful about exactly where I am, rather than agonizing over the upcoming day's adventures, and any events out of my control.

Mindfulness prepares you to deal with predictable events that can be extremely stressful, even when you're energized and ready to deal with them. While attending college in Washington, D.C., I was mugged early one evening by a rather macabre attacker, with one hook hand, wearing a mask and a hooded jacket. His two accomplices kept watch, and he pinned me to the wall of a house just feet from the sidewalk. Placing the hook under my throat, he growled a low noise and stared into my eyes. At first overwhelmed, I couldn't think straight or even scream. Somehow I decided this was not how my life would end, and resolved to survive. I mentally scrambled to remember self-defense tactics while trying to relax and breathe. I stared intently into his eyes, never losing focus, and shortly the residents of the house heard the commotion and opened the door. The muggers fled, and although shaken I was relieved I'd managed to remain composed. I then vowed to learn more effective self-defense techniques!

My consulting schedule frequently takes me to Paris, New York, Mexico City—cities renowned for many qualities, including their noise, traffic, and pollution. It helps to find creative ways to alleviate travel related stress. In each of those cities, I have found small parks and gardens that offer a tranquil respite, if only for a thirty-minute walk between meetings. Museums and even the lobbies of luxury hotels can provide solace for a frazzled traveler eager to focus on relaxation and breathing, before heading out to explore the city again.

Conversing with children forces us to be mindful, thanks to their natural curiosity. For example, when my little sister senses that I'm not giving her my complete attention, she will query me relentlessly until she is assured that I am focusing on her. The reward is often a pearl of wisdom generated by her inquisitive mind, which I would have missed if I had continued my scattered thinking about all the things I needed to accomplish over the next few hours.

For two decades now, I have been practicing a relaxation technique so effective that I now need only visualize the scene that provoked this state of mindfulness. I imagine myself on a remote stretch of beach, half immersed in the water, lying on my back on the warm sand. With each incoming wave, I feel energized and relaxed, while each outgoing wave carries away my stress and pain. By simply closing my eyes and lying on the floor, while paying attention to my breathing, I can feel the same therapeutic effect of that memorable day.

Sarah Weldon
Director of Strategic Partnerships and
Investor Outreach for Growthink
Los Angeles, California

✳ From the Author ✳

I WROTE THIS BOOK to share what I consider, the most important aspect of martial arts, sports, and activity—mindfulness. Mindfulness is that continuing, never ending, constant awareness. All martial artists no matter what style they practice, eventually get to a point where they learn to understand and cultivate this concept in order to reach the next level.

Anybody can throw a punch or a kick, but doing it mindfully is another thing. Relaxing and focusing all of your power and energy is an art. Mindfulness cultivates that art. Mindfulness is not inborn, but is always available to you. First you must learn the concept, and then you must practice it.

After you learn the concept of mindfulness, share it with your friends. As they become mindful there will be less arguing and conflict. When they share mindfulness with their acquaintances, peace of mind and harmony will spread to everyone, everywhere.

When we get caught up in our busy lives we forget our roots. My martial arts training began at the age of eleven. I studied in Asia and trained in a dojo that required strict discipline and self-control. There was no room for ego. If I didn't remain mindful of my stance, my Asian master promptly reminded me by taking me to the floor. After a year of training six nights a week for two hours a night, I was able to remain relaxed and focused throughout the training session. This is where I began to understand mindfulness. Mindfulness allows you to alter your activation levels at will so that you can relax and yet still be aware of your surroundings.

Recently, every time I boarded an airplane my heart raced. My doctor called it tachycardia. It was not that I was fearful of a crash; my anxiety was driven by thoughts of missing my connection or being late for a speaking engagement. While on long flights, I worked on my laptop computer, and I thought I was being productive. Even then, I experienced heart palpitations because I was worried that the battery to my computer might run down. I would type furiously without a bathroom break so I could get in as much writing as I could out of my two-hour flight. My work ethic spurred my compulsive nature. I forgot all about the mind/body connection, and mindfulness was no longer in my vocabulary.

When my laptop battery finally died, rather than let my mind wander and enjoy the flight, I would switch gears and force myself to spend idle moments preparing for my presentations. Takeoffs and landings were spent planning anecdotes for upcoming speeches. Sometimes, I would design karate combinations for my cardiokickboxing seminars. To me, idle thoughts were a non-productive waste of time. Talking with a fellow passenger seemed frivolous. Making the most out of every moment was more constructive.

Writing articles, books, and presenting every weekend became an ego trip. When I finally took the time to visit my dentist, he asked me about my rapid heartbeat. He suggested I visit the emergency room immediately. When I did, they found that my heart was racing at 150 beats per minute and occasionally would lose its rhythm. The doctors diagnosed an atrial fibrillation. I remained hospitalized for three days while physicians tried to figure out the cause.

They asked me if I was taking drugs or drinking too much coffee, but I knew what the problem was. My in-laws were visiting for the weekend, I was preparing for a race, and I was trying to get my writing career off the ground. I had too many irons in the fire and I was not coping. I had not recognized my own symptoms of stress, and I was overwhelmed. I lost my mindfulness.

Rather than mindfully experiencing the present moment on the plane, I focused on future fears. At first, I assumed my racing heart was normal and that everyone experienced preflight jitters. I soon became concerned that if my travel schedule increased, and my heart kept racing, I would suffer adrenal overload. Ironically, at the time, the topic of my speaking engagement at the time was "Relaxation of the Mind/Body."

Because mindfulness brings about total awareness it will teach you to recognize symptoms of anxiety. My symptom was a racing heart and shallow rapid breathing, and my eyes took on a driven gaze. Rather than enjoying a relaxed moment, I portrayed an image of unnecessary intensity. Fortunately I recognized my condition for what it was and through mindful practice was able to do something about it.

I credit my early martial arts experience with saving my life. When doctors could not explain my tachycardia and arrhythmia, I chose to return to my martial arts roots to provide a cure. I summoned the relaxed focus I learned in the dojo. Recollecting the power and energy present in my early training brought the stability back into my life that I had lost. Now each time I throw a punch or kick, or practice mindfulness, my mind is once again clear. I know now that stress provokes my arrhythmia. Mindfulness is the cure.

Sometimes mindfulness is simply focusing on the proper cues. Herb Perez, a Tae Kwon Do Olympic Gold Medalist is one of the most awesome fighters I have ever watched. But sometimes even a fighter of Herb's caliber needs a change of focus. I met Herb at the Taekwondo World Cup in Colorado Springs in 1986. I was the sports psychologist/physiologist for the U.S. Team. Herb was having trouble sleeping the night before his bouts and he came to me for advice. Knowing how Herb trained I told him it's not the amount of sleep that you get the night before your fight, it's the quality of sleep you get the *weeks* before." With the pressure of worrying over sleep off, Herb was able to win gold medals at the World Cup, Pan-Am Games, and finally at the 1992 Olympic Games in Barcelona.

I certainly will not take any credit for Herb's outstanding performances but I will suggest that sometimes you need to take a look at what you're doing, and how you're doing it. Then, if you're mindful, nothing can stand in your way.

I took the benefits of that early martial arts training into other areas of my life—tennis, cycling, and academics. The discipline and mindfulness required in the dojo truly enhanced every area of my life.

❋ Preface ❋

To possess the total integration of your mind and body requires you to be relaxed and focused. I call this mind/body. You know how to relax—or at least you think you do. Your muscles are stiff. Perhaps you are trying too hard. When you attempt to relax, you are unsuccessful because you are thinking too much.

Think of only one thing. Whether you pay attention to your breathing, your heart rate, or your spouse, you are experiencing mindfulness. Mindfulness has everything to do with relaxation and focus.

Mind/body fitness is all about awareness. Your friends may choose to play tennis or jog. You need to find what is good for you. Although affiliation and camaraderie make activity fun, it is more important that you perform your workout on your terms. Do what you love. Do what is right for your mind/body.

You know when a movement or thought is right for your body or your mind, and you know when it is wrong. Your mind/body will rebel against inappropriate movements or thoughts. Perhaps at first you enjoyed running and anti-inflammatory medication dulled any discomfort you may have experienced. Then the pain and confusion became stronger than any sedative. Soon your knees and hips told you to walk. Finally, stationary cycling became your non-impact activity of choice.

Group exercise leaders crank up their music so students are distracted from discomfort. They count rhythmically and entice their charges to ignore pain. Every once in a while, an insightful instructor turns off the music. The students listen to their bodies instead of chaos. At this point, there is nothing to dull their sensations. These students are mindful of their movement without distraction.

Be mindful during your activities. Practice martial arts or go bowling, cycling, or running. Whatever your choice, if you are relaxed and focused, you are practicing mindfulness. Rather than fretting about your bowling score or how many calories you are burning, remain in the present. Do not fear victory or anticipate success. Play. Immerse yourself in your action. Associate with your activity. Become fully involved in whatever you are doing with no second guesses.

Dissociation, the opposite of association, may be considered mindful exercise. Sometimes when practicing, martial artists, long distance cyclists, and marathon runners dissociate their minds from pain. Instead, they let their minds wander to grocery lists, dinner, or building their fortunes. Tibetan monks dissociate to achieve altered states of consciousness. You too dissociate every day of your life, for example, by doodling and daydreaming.

Burned out athletes find mind/body training revitalizing. Mind/body activities can include pilates, taijiquan, yoga, and individualized programs provided in this book. You can use mind/body techniques to warmup and cooldown during athletics. Because in these activities you do not pound the pavement, mind/body training appeals to those fearful of high-intensity physical training routines. Mind/body practice results in other benefits as well, including stress management, improved concentration, and enhanced discipline.

❋ Introduction ❋

Your Body and Your Brain

MERICANS ARE SEARCHING for a magic bullet. There are more get-in-shape pills, gimmicks, and gadgets than ever, yet Americans are fatter, lazier, and more out of shape now than at any other time in human history. Martial arts classes overflow with desperate, overweight men and women who are willing to do anything to lose weight. Even high intensity cardio-kickboxing classes that can burn as much as 500 calories in an hour do not affect the students' overfed paunches.

It is true, you need to eat well to train in the martial arts, but you also need to eat for the right reasons. If you eat because you are tired, bored, anxious, or excited, then your focus is not on your well-being, it is on the food. Mindfulness will teach you how to focus on yourself instead of focusing on food. Instead of eating when you are anxious or excited, you will learn to do relaxation strategies. If you are tired or bored, you will learn to increase your activation or performance level. To get fit, you must also use your mind. Your body will follow.

One of the main reasons many martial artists are out of shape is lack of proper exercise caused by convenience. Today we have drive-through everything, including weddings and funeral parlors. TV remote controls and automatic garage door openers add additional ease to your life. Ease, however should not be your priority. A mind/body connection will provide you with the motivation to get off and stay off the couch. You will learn about yourself and how to enjoy your body.

Included in this book are various mind/body exercise protocols. Just choose a program and begin. That is how easy it is to get started.

This book is not just about getting fit. It is about learning to use your mind. Mindfulness is not a new idea. Maharishi brought relaxed concentration to the United States from India and popularized it as meditation. Chinese martial artists have been practicing various mind/body strategies for centuries. Native Americans, Africans, and Asians have found natural ways of moving to connect their bodies and minds. The concepts of balance, yin and yang, and oneness with the universe have been around for a long time. No one has all the answers, but if you look you can learn a little bit from every culture.

In the 1970s, Transcendental Meditation (TM) classes became popular in the United States. Thousands of Americans signed up for such classes seeking mindfulness. Some soon found that seated meditation was difficult and boring. Practitioners would often fall asleep in mid-trance. Many programs that promise mindfulness have come and gone, such as progressive relaxation, autogenic training, hypnosis, and imagery. Although there is nothing inherently wrong with these strategies, Americans seem to be searching for something more. Mind/body fitness is different. It combines breathing, punching, kicking, or pedaling with mindful contemplation. It allows you to experience the moment.

The fitness/martial arts industry can be a trendy one. In the past few years, we have seen an explosion of fitness trends that include spinning, pilates, yoga, and taijiquan to name a few. With each new fad, there are new fitness-fad-fraud gurus who try to separate you from your hard-earned money. *Mind/Body Fitness* will provide you with information that will allow you to make informed decisions about your martial arts/mindfulness program.

- ► What martial arts/mindfulness program is right for you?
- ► What do you look for in a martial arts/mindfulness instructor?
- ► How can you build your own martial arts/mindfulness program?

All of these questions and more are answered. You will learn to develop your own mind/body program and center around it any martial arts, sport, or fitness activity. Your mind/body experience will become personalized to your individual needs and goals.

Let us try something right now! Inhale a deep breath from your diaphragm and raise your arms over your head. Exhale, lower your arms, and allow all of your muscles to relax. Continue to inhale up, exhale down as long as you like. Relax and focus only on your breath. With each exhalation, allow your body to relax until you are not thinking about your arms or your breath. At this point, there is no thought, and you are experiencing mindfulness.

Why Mind/Body? Why Mindfulness?

The secret to success in martial arts, sports, fitness, and even life is mindfulness. Because it has no rules, mindfulness can be practiced at work or play. Mindfulness is simply the art of paying attention. Paying attention to your body, your breath, and your brain. Within the martial arts world, the fitness industry and sports arenas, mindfulness is dubbed mind/body. Thus mindfulness and mind/body are one in the same.

Mind/body fitness is the newest quest for those athletes seeking something extra. Mind/body workouts provide martial artists as well as fitness enthusiasts with a well-rounded, mind/body program. At first, tuning into your body can be a chore. Silence can be intimidating so we fill our lives with radios, televisions, and other audio diversions. Sitting in silence can be uncomfortable. Yet, if you learn to tune into your own internal "TV," you will not believe what is in there. You will begin to see the excitement that we have been covering up for years with mindless noise. Soon you will not be able to imagine what it was like to train without mindfulness.

Each chapter of this book provides you with the tools and motivation to enjoy your own mind/body program. The most difficult part of this training, however, is to remember to practice it. It is easy to get caught up in your own activity. Each mind/body program gives you easy-to-follow drills and reminders so you can work mindfulness into your martial arts, sports, and fitness programs.

Mindfulness can improve every aspect of your martial arts training and performance, since your sport/fitness activity is based on motivation, activation, and concentration to reach your mind/body best. Whether your goal is to lose weight; gain muscle; increase speed, flexibility, or endurance; or improve health, your first step begins in your brain. Once you begin, you can apply mindfulness to every aspect of your life.

Introduction to Mindfulness

Recently, while I was on an airplane, I watched a video ad that suggested "what if you did not have to worry about the stock market, reading faxes, and returning emails." For a moment I was intrigued, thinking perhaps that I was going to hear of a new mindfulness strategy that would allow transcendence from the everyday busy lifestyles that we all encounter. Rather, the commercial turned out to be an advertisement proposing that if we cannot spend our waking hours committing to more and more, then we are capable of less.

I feel the opposite is true. Simplicity is the answer. Rather than grandeur and extravagance, we need to master the basics. We need to whittle away the superfluous and refine and reshape our lifestyles.

Less is more. If you look at those that possess a mastery of their craft you will see movement to simplicity. A fighter who masters one or two powerful attacks cannot be beaten. A player who makes fewer mistakes has streamlined her strokes.

To return to the basics and focus on simplicity is not easy. Simplicity is not the nature of our culture; variety is usually a welcome distraction. Practicing mindfulness requires discipline and perseverance. You must focus on your movements, pay attention to the nuances, and refine the subtleties in order to sharpen your technique.

Whether you are a martial artist, professional athlete, or a weekend warrior, mindfulness is your reward beyond athletic prowess. It will teach you self-awareness that will provide you with the proper feedback to get to the next level. If you raise the bar and challenge yourself, you will find that you can achieve more than you ever dreamed possible.

Mindfulness will improve your martial arts and fitness levels, and it will enhance your confidence and mental development. Just as it requires training to improve your martial arts, it takes practice to enhance your mindfulness. You must learn to use your brain in a way similar to athletic training. Mindfulness is performing martial arts, physical skills, or fitness exercises with an inward focus on attention.

This internal focus is non-judgmental and requires no goal setting. You must focus your breath and monitor your muscles. Do not be concerned with results. Every act should be an end in itself.

You cannot learn mindfulness through osmosis from a book. Practice is your answer. Later on in this book you will learn that mindfulness is a combination of your breathing, movement, and mindset. Your movements should be graceful yet controlled. Mindfulness enhances your concentration, speed, and force. Relaxation and concentration are key to speed, and if your speed is adequate, your strength increases your force. With improved concentration, speed, and force in combination, your power and effectiveness will increase.

Mindfulness is an overall approach to your martial arts training, exercise, and life. You can use mindfulness not only to enhance your awareness, concentration, and performance, but also to live each day fully. Follow your personal mind/body mission statement. Do not expect results overnight. Progress gradually. Mindfulness is a single-minded focus. First learn to relax and then work on improving power, effectiveness, and life in general.

Maybe you think there is no need for you to pursue a mind/body program. If this is true then maybe you need to re-evaluate where you are in the scheme of things. Everyone can benefit from a mind/body program. Control your mind and discipline your body. Seek a balance between your mind and body. Try it. The results may surprise you. If you think mind/body is not right for you, let it go. Soon you will return.

Mindfulness is based on your emotions, thoughts, and feelings and how they affect your health, fitness, and martial arts performance. Look at yourself as a whole person and acknowledge that your mind programs your body. Your mind influences your body more than you imagine. Each thought that you think influences each step you take.

Mindfulness helps you cope with stress and anxiety. Place emphasis on the quality of your life, rather than a dog-eat-dog survival mode. Develop confidence to make positive changes. For the first time, take charge of your performance and your health. Know that you are in control and that no one is looking over your shoulder telling you what to do.

Using this Book

Mind/Body Fitness is a book dedicated to teach, guide, and assist you to achieve optimal well-being, health, fitness, and sports enhancement through a balance of physical activity and mindfulness.

Embraced by medical professionals and supported by scientific research, mind/body strategies facilitate numerous health benefits. Within a mind/body program, "mind" activities such as meditation, visualization, prayer, and breathing techniques integrate with "body" (physical activities) to promote balance and focus in your life.

My mind/body programs are designed to meet your needs and goals, to heighten awareness of your physical, mental, and emotional health, and to provide inspiration for your fitness and sports performance.

Within the content of this book you may perceive apparent paradoxes. Look beneath the words. At certain times you may react differently to the same situation. There certainly is no black and white.

- ‣ Music may be a distraction one day and motivation the next.
- ‣ You may strive to reach a goal yet remain mindfully in the present.
- ‣ Adhering to a strict schedule does not crush your spontaneity or mindfulness.
- ‣ You may be productive and mindfully creative simultaneously.
- ‣ You can be exhilarated and mindful at the same time.
- ‣ You can fight to win or just fight your best without losing focus.

Although these seem opposite, all may be accomplished. You can do them all. This book can show you the way. Read it with an open mind. You will come to understand that there is a *yin/yang*, Zen-like quality to everything you do.

✳ Acknowledgements ✳

My mind/body experience has been shaped by my immediate family, my martial arts instructors, my friends, and my students. My mother and father raised me in the Catholic faith, but encouraged me to enroll in meditation and martial arts. My instructors provided me with the groundwork to make my own decisions about mindfulness. My friends shared their mind/body triumphs and tragedies. My students diligently pursued their mindful strategies of choice.

Once again I would like to thank YMAA for their friendly direction, powerful information, and exemplary publishing system. And a special thanks to wordsmith Sharon Rose who spent countless hours adding her valuable insight and wonderful writing style to *Mind/Body Fitness*.

Traditional Mind/Body

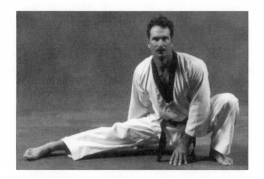

✳ Traditional Mind/Body ✳

Being Attentive Reduces Stress

M OST AMERICANS do not take the debilitating effects of stress seriously. You know that it is important to quit smoking and exercise, but do you take the time to regularly relax? When you finally take the time to relax, do you find it difficult because you are trying too hard? If you try too hard, you will tense, and relaxation will not happen. It is like trying to sleep. Let go or you will peek at your alarm every hour. Mindfulness will help you to relax. Relaxation can begin in your body or your mind: The choice is yours.

During extended periods of unrelenting stress, your norepinephrine and cortisol levels remain elevated. These are your stress hormones. They contribute to high blood pressure, abdominal weight gain, insulin resistance, and a fatty lipid profile. Combine these physical effects of stress with too many calories and limited activity, and you have the beginnings of cardiovascular disease. Stress also affects your immune system by over-secreting cortisol, which can increase your chances for bouts of asthma, skin problems, irritable bowel syndrome, and arthritis. Your "B" immune cells that normally fight off infection decrease when you are under stress. During stressful times this immune response contributes to increased colds and flu. If you learn to recognize the symptoms of your stress, you can mindfully curb the harmful side effects.

Recent research has demonstrated that stress causes impaired memory and is associated with brain cell loss. When stressed, you have problems with brain function.

Additionally, stress also decreases fertility. For example, often couples put unnecessary pressure on themselves to conceive a child, but they cannot do so. Yet when they finally give up their attempts, they conceive because the pressure was taken off. Relax, do not try so hard, and things will come to you. Relaxed concentration leads to mindfulness, and mindfulness enhances your performance.

Different thresholds of stress create boiling points for some and enjoyment for others. There is no exact measure of how much stress one can handle, but it is important to deal with your feelings of anger and hostility to remain healthy. Do not allow negative feelings to ferment. Deal with negativity immediately. Choose your coping strategy, and decide exactly how to proceed.

When times get tough, try a combination of humor and optimism. Awareness of your stress levels can keep it from gaining a toehold and uprooting your mindfulness.

Not all mind/body activities require physical relaxation, although relaxation is a side effect of it. For example, if you practice repetitive punches, or pedal a bike, you will be surprised to find mindfulness. Punching methodically, and pedaling at an easy cadence are naturally relaxing. Think back to peaceful times. What were you doing? Were you mindful? Go there now.

There are many simple ways to relax. When stress gets the best of you and you have had enough, look out of the window, doodle, or daydream. These are automatic mind/body strategies that seem to be instinctive and may help remove some tension and allow you to relax. During times of increased tension choose activities where you are controlled, relaxed, and focused. For example singing is a natural path to relaxation and mindfulness. Singing slows neural impulses and calms brain activity as well as regulates your breathing and heart rate. When you are stressed, try humming your favorite song instead of counting to ten.

Your various activities are governed by your brain. Left brain activities draw on your logic center while right brain activities draw on your creative center. Right brain activities include artwork, playing musical instruments, and riding your bike. You practice imagery from you right brain. Your right brain sees the whole picture. Alpha brain wave patterns produced by such activities pull you into a state of relaxed concentration or mindfulness. My wife, Danese, was a computer science major and is logical and very analytical. I am right-brained and am more concerned with introspection, form, physiology, and emotion. See if you can figure out whether you are left-brained, right-brained, or a little of both. Understanding where you are helps you to change if need be. This is mindfulness.

Mindfulness allows you to immerse yourself in activity. Because you become immersed in what you are doing, mindfulness decreases stress, boredom, and anxiety. Mindfulness exists in the moment.

Mindful activity reduces stress, tension, anxiety, and depression. It increases your vigor and helps you to think clearly. Physical activity gathers pent-up, fight-or-flight energy and turns it into a homerun blast or a front kick through a heavy bag. When you practice physical and mindful activity, your body becomes calm, relaxed, and refreshed, and your mood will remain mindful.

Mindful exercise also decreases burnout and increases your self-confidence. Those who practice mindful exercise regularly view their jobs as less stressful than those who do not practice mindful exercise. Mindful individuals find that they are more productive and can concentrate better than their sedentary counterparts.

Your body was designed for mindful activity. Movement is play, not something at which you have to work. Everyone has a set-point for happiness. As an example, let us look at joyfulness on a continuum from one to ten. Perhaps a colleague of yours may hover around eight, while you may be stuck at three. Boosting your level of happiness requires mindfulness, awareness of your activation, and concentration. Such a level of mindfulness will allow you to change. Mindful martial arts training and exercise promote an endorphin release—a morphine-like substance that relieves pain, and enhances your capacity for joy astronomically, helping to raise your set point level.

Characteristics of Mindfulness

Answer honestly the following questions:

- ▸ Are you spending time working toward your health and fitness?
- ▸ Are you mindful of your exercise?
- ▸ Do pleasures have to be justified or earned?

Think for a moment about your answers. You must realize that you do not have to wait for a reward for exercising or training in martial arts. Rather than thinking about what you are going to do next, enjoy each moment of your workout for its own sake. Otherwise, you will probably quit.

Put yourself in the moment during your workouts and take them seriously. Set workout goals and do not worry about instant gratification. Results will take as long as they take. Allow your workouts to be an enjoyable, healthy escape from the real world. To do this, be familiar with your surroundings, wear comfortable clothing, and compete only against yourself. Turn off your Walkman or cardio-theatre. Begin with a deep cleansing breath and warm up by performing your activity at a slow pace. While training, your mind may stray from your movement. Try to stay mindful of the movement; exist in the moment, and gently remind yourself to focus.

Pay attention to how you schedule your time. If you have too much to do and not enough time in which to do it, you will be stressed and feel out of control. Remain in control and enjoy a sense of purpose. You will be more resistant to stress. The last thing you need when you have got a lot going on in your life is to get sick. Illness can be like a warning signal; it may be the only thing that will slow you down. If you stay in control you can avoid such situations. Keep yourself healthy, get enough sleep, eat right, take a multi-vitamin, avoid too much caffeine and alcohol, and workout every other day. Exercise is a form of stress management. It also helps to prevent cardiovascular disease, high blood pressure, diabetes, osteoporosis, obesity, anxiety, and depression. Activity provides a break in your busy day and helps you feel relaxed and refreshed as well as improving the quality of your sleep.

Some people work out to improve their mindfulness as well as their physical condition. Many search for mindfulness through the ultimate mind/body experience. They "spin" stationary bikes or practice pilates or yoga; others turn to martial arts, taijiquan, cardio-kickboxing, or forms of aerobic exercise to help them achieve mindfulness. Some people follow fitness gurus who claim if you follow their teachings you will find "the way." In fact, these gurus are throwbacks from the Maharishi days of the early 1970s. It seems that every twenty years or so, cycles repeat and, in reality, there is nothing new under the sun.

Although there is no single mind/body strategy, mindfulness is worth pursuing. I have yet to meet anyone who has achieved a constant state of mindfulness. That is okay, though, because mindfulness is taking one moment at a time. It is a process. When things are right, you know it. You want that moment to last forever. Prolong it. Remain relaxed and focused.

I spoke to a taijiquan master and asked if he knew anyone who was mindful one hundred percent of the time. He first spoke of his own experience. He meditates four hours a day, from 4:00 A.M. until 6:00 A.M. and then from 1:00 P.M. until 3:00 P.M. This man wrote more than thirty books and earned a Ph.D. in electrical engineering. I was amazed by his discipline and asked him about his progress towards mindfulness. He told me he had not reached perpetual mindfulness and that he did not know of anyone who has. He said, "if someone has reached this state, he is living far away in the mountains."

In my own experience, I found that repetitive activities help me achieve mindfulness for brief periods of time. Martial arts, cycling, meditating, skipping rope, and walking are mindful activities for me. While my body is busy pedaling, my mind is free to be mindful or to simply focus on breathing. When I focus on my breath, my body relaxes. I have not reached a state of perpetual mindfulness, but at least I am experiencing it more often.

Meditation or prayer may not provoke mindfulness outright, but they can help. Because we are all individuals, no one person can say his or her way is the only way to mindfulness. It is important to find your own way. Pedaling a bicycle across America or meditating four hours a day will not ensure that you will live mindfully. Some gurus may suggest that repetitive activity or repeating a mantra is all you need to do.

They say repetitive practice will provide the discipline and perseverance to find yourself totally. If it were that easy, everyone would do it. Yet we do not all do it.

Misinformation and misperception of fitness enthusiasts and athletes is rampant. Sure, there are a few brain cell-challenged athletes who perpetuate the stereotype. However, some of the smartest people I know are athletes. They are paid millions to play, and "play" is a perfect activity during which to practice mindfulness. These individuals understand that if you lose your focus, you lose your game.

Professional athletics require extraordinary mindfulness. Making a game-winning free-throw, "threading a needle" with a touchdown pass, and breaking a couple of cinder blocks is not easy. Mindfulness makes it possible.

Activity increases oxygen to your brain and stimulates your creativity. Some studies suggest that movement will increase your alertness, reaction time, and decision-making skills. So next time you see a professional athlete or martial artist, pay him or her the respect due to such an athlete. They understand the mind/body connection and—who knows—they may turn out to be a prototype of you.

Choosing Your Mind/Body Strategy

So far we have discussed a few physical strategies to enhance mindfulness, but what about spiritual and psychological techniques? There are dozens of such techniques practiced today. Taijiquan, meditation, and prayer are examples of spiritual techniques that may help you on your quest for single-minded focus.

The difficulty, however, lies in discovering which mind/body strategy works best for you. For example:

> - Some folks were raised as followers from childhood to death. Their eyes never waver, and there are no questions. They are certain of their future and remain disciplined in their faith. They have no time or inclination for mindfulness.

▸ Others, however, spend years searching for mindfulness. They delve into different mind/body techniques and, after years of trial and error, they find their answers and develop a single-minded focus.

▸ Still others spend their lives adding and deleting to an amorphous profile, constantly refining their strategies. They combine physical and psychological techniques while learning the secrets to mindful living. They improve their focus and continue their path to increased mindfulness.

Perhaps you are in the last of the above-mentioned situations. Maybe you have sampled different techniques, yet still have something missing. Maybe you tried meditation—for awhile, that seemed to work, but not for long. You realized there was more. Your search for enhanced mindfulness is never ending. Perhaps that is why you chose this book.

Develop what works for you. Choose bits and pieces of the strategies presented in this book and create your own mindfulness program. There is no reason to flounder in a sea of misinformation. A guru may say "my way or the highway." Meditation instructors promise if you pay just $499, you will reach enlightenment in five to eight years. Achieving mindfulness begins today, and the truth is that there is no single way to do it.

As I mentioned earlier, some individuals substitute drugs and alcohol as alternatives for mindfulness. These substances cannot provide lasting effects. Do not be fooled, however; activities like martial arts, meditation, or riding a bicycle do not provide lasting effects either. Repeating a mantra or fitness training can help, but when you stop, your problems will soon return. You need a gentle reminder every few minutes of every day to be mindful. Mindfulness is ongoing twenty-four hours a day everyday. It begins when you awaken and continues until you sleep. You get better and better with practice, so practice whenever you can.

The following checklist can be used to help you remain mindful. As you begin to practice mindfulness, ask yourself these questions every hour.

QUESTIONS FOR PRACTICE

---

1. Are you tired, bored, or too excited?

2. Is your focus of concentration appropriate to your task?

3. Is your activity thought-provoking or non-productive?

4. Is there an ultimate goal to your activity?

5. Is your breathing from your chest or from your abdomen?

6. Are your thoughts scattered or focused?

7. Is your body tight or relaxed?

8. Are you focusing on the nostalgia of the past?

9. Are you worried about the future?

10. Are you afraid of failure or success?

After you have answered the above questions, manipulate your environment to achieve mindfulness. Mindfulness is the reward for your efforts. Do not try too hard, though, because that will bring tension. Give yourself permission to enjoy yourself. If you are afraid to fail, you will.

Practicing mindfulness is a daily ritual. Although you may be mired in fear of the future or worried about something over which you have no control, you are doing better than you think. List the positives and pay attention to them.

PAY ATTENTION TO...

---

1. Your energy level.

2. Your relaxed mindset.

3. Your ability to focus.

4. Your productivity.

5. Your ability to enjoy yourself.

Please keep in mind, however, that there are frauds peddling mind/body wares on every corner. For your own sake, learn to recognize self-proclaimed mind/body gurus that will separate you from your money and nothing else.

BE AWARE IF...

---

1. They say they know all of the answers

2. They are too sure of themselves.

3. They say, "it is easy" and "anyone can do it."

4. They are moody.

5. They are irritable (perhaps when they think you are not watching).

6. They are unfriendly and aloof.

7. They try to appear as if they are always in control.

8. They are emotionless.

9. They say that their way is the only way.

10. They are obsessive, overweight, or controlling.

It is important that you learn to trust yourself. Your mind/body program should meet your needs, not the needs that someone else tells you to meet.

Benefits of Mind/Body

Mindfulness in your martial art and physical activity affects your mental and emotional processes. Practicing mindfulness will allow you to think more clearly, be more creative, increase your brain cell growth, improve your self-esteem, decrease depression, and improve your short-term memory. It has always been a wonder to me why people do not get off of the couch sooner. To me, it is more excruciating to sit than it is to enjoy mindful activity.

It is not scientifically known why mind/body programming helps you to think clearly and improve your memory, but it may be related to an increased body temperature and the improved oxygenation of your brain.

We humans were not biologically designed to be sedentary. Your body functions best when you move. Take children, for example. They cannot sit still for a minute. Somehow, in our overfed, underactive society, we have lost the desire to move. The less we move, the less we oxygenate our blood and the more stagnant we become.

In addition to the benefits you get from moving, mind/body fitness programming provides several other benefits.

1. Mindful exercise decreases stress. Let me explain how this works. First, exercise is a stressor so it teaches you to deal with other stresses. Second, mind/body workouts help you to relax so you are less stressed when you complete your program.
2. Since you are biologically designed to move, couch potatoes generally become depressed due largely to their sedentary lifestyle. Thus, mind/body training is a natural antidepressant. Movement is stimulating, and physical activity provides you with energy. The harder you train, the more energy you will have. It seems like a paradox, but it works.
3. Mindful exercise improves self-confidence because exercise increases bodily attractiveness, strength, and muscular fitness.
4. Increased confidence provides you with energy and increased energy allows you to complete your mind/body program. It is an energetic cycle of completeness.
5. Although you may have heard the myths about "dumb jocks," regular mind/body exercise has been shown to spur the growth of new brain cells in laboratory animals. Exercise also prolongs the survival of brain cells. I do not know about you, but I can use all of the brain cells that I can get.
6. Faith is another type of mind/body training that can also increase health and longevity. More than 300 studies analyzed the effects of faith on healing. Seventy-five percent of these studies have shown that believing in God or a higher power is good for your health. Individuals that are deeply religious exhibit a longer life expectancy, quicker recovery, better quality of life, and lower rates of depression and substance abuse. Every culture has a belief in some sort of higher power; belief in it, it seems, is empowering.

A study at Dartmouth College revealed the best predictor of heart bypass survival rates was whether or not patients believed in God. It was found that six months after surgery, twelve percent of non-believers died yet one hundred percent of believers were still living. A Gallup survey found that ninety percent of Americans believe in God, sixty percent to seventy percent contend that faith can help people recover from illness, and forty-one percent say their faith has healed either mental or physical problems.

Although doctors rarely discuss religion with their patients, ninety-nine percent of physicians surveyed responded that faith or meditation aids in healing. Eighty percent of M.D.'s surveyed think that spiritual concepts should be part of a doctor's training. In America, only one-third of the medical schools offer courses in spirituality and healing.

The Mind/Body Connection for Stress Management

Stress is anything that stimulates you and increases your activation. Life without stimulation would be incredibly dull and boring. However, life with too many stimuli becomes unpleasant and tiring and ultimately damages your health.

- Stress happens when your survival or health is threatened, when you are under pressure, or when you experience a challenge. When you are under stress, adrenaline is released, and you experience symptoms that your body is preparing to fight-or-flight.
- Internal stress comes from worrying about events beyond your control, from a harried approach to life, or from an addictive-type enjoyment of stress.
- Life stress occurs when your work or living environment causes anxiety. Noise, crowding, pollution, dirt, and other distractions can lead to life stress.
- Burnout is a type of stress that builds up over a long period. This happens when you push yourself too hard or when you forget to use proper time management skills.

If you can remember the following ten tips, you will be able to manage stress.

TIPS FOR STRESS MANAGEMENT

---

1. The stress you experience is largely under your control.

2. Stress comes from a variety of different sources.

3. Short-term stress is situational.

4. A certain amount of stress keeps you invigorated.

5. Too much stress hampers your performance.

6. Breathing and other anxiety management techniques help you handle stress.

7. Chronic stress comes from a gradual buildup.

8. Chronic, high level stress can cause illness.

9. Chronic stress is best managed by changes in your lifestyle and attitude.

10. Understand the causes of your stress, and then channel it to improve your performance.

Stress enters your life through your senses. You can also use your senses to relax. Make time in your life where you can mindfully enjoy relaxation through your senses. The following are ways that we can relax by experiencing with our senses.

- Touch. Hug a friend or a pet. Get a massage. Both massage and hugging have been proven to reduce tension. If you calm your body, your mind will follow.
- Sound. Relax and enjoy the sound of rustling leaves, surf rolling, or raindrops falling. Listen to relaxing music such as baroque music played at sixty beats per minute. Enjoy silence. You will even find that the sound of silence during meditation is magical.
- Smell. Some people find comfort in relaxing scents: lavender, vanilla, rose, and jasmine to name a few. Some may find the aroma of baked goods brings back memories of a warm comfortable kitchen.
- Taste. Comfort foods can increase seratonin in your brain, which helps you to relax. These include carbohydrates—breads, cereals, grains, fruits, and vegetables. Eating such foods when you are stressed can help you relax.

▸ Sight. Peering into your child's bedroom while he is fast asleep or delighting in the antics of a playful puppy can awaken profound feelings of relaxation and joyfulness.

Traditional Mind/Body Workouts

Mind/body is not just adding a meditative warmup or taijiquan cool down to your training. Characteristics of mind/body training include:

MIND/BODY TRAINING STRATEGIES

---

1. Adjust your activation level so you are not bored or agitated.

2. Relax through your entire mind/body experience.

3. Actively focus on the proper cues to enjoy alpha brain wave activity.

4. Possess a non-competitive attitude.

5. Never try too hard. Expend efforts that increase, not decrease, your energy.

6. Exist in the moment. Do not worry about the past or wonder what the future holds.

7. Do not judge your performance.

8. Consciously associate or dissociate from your activity.

9. Focus on your breath. Your breath may be the focal point of your training.

10. Pay attention to your posture. Are your shoulders back? Is your spine neutral, and is your chest is open during your entire activity?

Examples of traditional mind/body training include yoga, taijiquan, progressive relaxation, autogenic training, and some martial arts. Depending on your fitness level, choose the training that appeals to you. For example, taijiquan improves balance, flexibility, and concentration in young and old alike. Yoga can improve your strength, flexibility, and reduce your stress levels. However, pilates and some forms of power yoga can be very vigorous. Below are several mind/body workouts for you to sample.

TAIJIQUAN (TAI CHI CHUAN). The word *taijiquan* translates into "supreme or grand ultimate fist." Its roots come from ancient China approximately four thousand years ago. Taijiquan originated from the Taoist (Daoist) school of thought and was practiced for self-defense and spiritual cultivation. Taijiquan is a relaxed and slow-moving meditation as well as an effective martial art. Practice of it can help center you and get you in touch with you body and mind. As you practice taijiquan you will become aware of your body's internal energy or qi (chi). Continued practice can result in smooth qi flow and good blood circulation. Taijiquan is based on the study of the yin and yang diagram, which represents a perfect balance between two opposing forces. Achieving this balance is a function of your qi: keeping an uninterrupted flow of qi promotes your physical and psychological well-being.

A variety of studies have demonstrated that taijiquan increases your balance and coordination. Results of a recent investigation demonstrated that taijiquan also increased aerobic capacity. Because of its graded, gentle increase in intensity, taijiquan is an ideal mind/body strategy for people of all ages, and it can be especially beneficial program for older adults. Taijiquan increases you balance by improving your proprioception (body awareness), thus making it a great tool for learning and practicing mindfulness—and for older adults, it decreases their chances of falling. Recent investigations involving older adults produced evidence that taijiquan helps lower blood pressure. Blood pressure reductions in older taijiquan participants have been found to be similar to subjects who participated in moderate-intensity aerobic exercise. Older adults who practice taijiquan daily show significant improvements in heart health and cardiovascular function. Taijiquan can be effective by itself or in addition to aerobic exercise. For example, taijiquan can be practiced along with a cardiovascular activity such as walking. Best of all, taijiquan is safe. Students of taijiquan are taught to be aware of their bodies and their physical limitations. Practitioners learn to maintain stable footing until they develop a firm "root" or connection to the earth.

Taijiquan movements are low impact. Rheumatoid arthritis patients who practiced taijiquan for ten weeks had no increase in joint symptoms in comparison with patients who were not involved in taijiquan. An instructor who is appropriately trained in the art should supervise students so as to monitor their postures and movements. What is nice about taijiquan is that anyone can do it; the instructor can modify the postures to accommodate the specific needs of your body.

QIGONG (CHI KUNG). *Qigong,* like taijiquan, has roots in ancient China. The practice of qigong is the study or understanding of your body's *qi.* Qigong in its narrowest sense is a series of exercises and meditations that promotes a healthy body and mind. Its study, however, goes well beyond the healing realm. The practice of qigong can help promote mindfulness and a connection to nature. When you practice qigong movements you stimulate energy pathways or meridians in your body that help your *qi* flow. Many of the movements are patterned after animals such as the monkey (agility), crane (steadiness), and tortoise (longevity). All of your movements are used to stimulate *qi* and generate powerful energy.

YOGA. *Yoga* is an eastern discipline that employs meditation, breathing, and physical exercise to connect the body and the mind. Yoga begins with your body and ends with your mind. By practicing breathing, twists, bends, balances, poses, postures, and movements, you develop discipline and self-control. The postures bring your body alive by promoting flexibility, strength, and power. Far Eastern yogis incorporate meditation and physical practice to reach altered states of consciousness. They develop a unique ability to focus their concentration to block pain and achieve extraordinary postures. Yoga practitioners do not see the mind and body as separate; they think of both as one. Science and common sense show the two have a direct effect on each other. A combination of yoga stretching and breathing brings about changes in your central nervous system as well as an increase in blood oxygenation and circulation. Yoga can be as strenuous as you want it to be. Some say you could get better exercise jogging, but yoga masters argue that jogging will not improve your mindfulness.

A recent study compared yoga to swimming in the area of stress reduction. It was found that they both reduced stress, but in men yoga also helped decrease anger. It was found that the breathing exercises practiced in yoga stimulate your vagus nerve, which is part of your peripheral nervous system. Such stimulation will slow your heart rate and decrease your arousal. Therefore, if you need to relax, yoga may be more beneficial for you than swimming.

Another study compared the differences between cycling and cycling/yoga training programs. The cycling-plus-yoga group had fewer cardiac events and lived longer than the cycling-only group.

Some of the meditative yoga postures were found to decrease the pain associated with angina. What that means is that heart patients were able to handle their angina pain more effectively after yoga training then before they practiced yoga. Yoga has also been shown to reduce symptoms of chronic obstructive pulmonary disease (COPD). If you do decide to use yoga as part of your mind/body program, ask your instructor if he or she can measure your progress. They should provide you with pre- and post-tests in flexibility, strength, balance, anxiety, tension, blood pressure, and quality of life.

MEDITATION. *Meditation* begins in your mind and ends with your body. By freeing your mind from beta (conscious, anxiety-producing) activity, you learn to relax in an alpha state. Stress sometimes becomes so prevalent in our lives that it is difficult to enjoy the alpha state, which is characterized by relaxation and concentration. Meditation will release tension from your muscles, calm your emotions, and reduce anxiety. Remember, though, that meditation is a skill that takes practice. Once you begin to practice meditation, however, it snowballs, and you get better and better at it.

Meditation is not a competition. Enjoy the process. Do not try to solve your problems during meditation. Instead, take a break from worrying and planning. Meditation is your vacation from the world. Energy accrued during meditation can then funnel into the rest of your life.

Meditation or mindfulness does not necessarily mean sitting cross-legged in a quiet room. Be mindful while you are driving, taking out the trash, or mowing the lawn. Mindfulness is a part of your every act, and any activity is a mindful exercise if you concentrate on the task you are performing. If you do meditate by sitting quietly in a room, carry the mindfulness you are experiencing into the next few minutes of your waking world. Although it may be difficult, try five minutes of walking or stationary cycling immediately following your sitting meditation. Concentrating on your rhythmic gait or pedal stroke will fuel your mindfulness.

There is little difference between your sitting meditation and your active mindfulness. Your alpha brain waves patterns will follow you through each endeavor. Your whole life can be a practice of meditation and mindfulness...if you let it.

PILATES. The founder of *pilates* as a child was a small and frail boy. To combat this, he started exercising and became a good boxer, skier, and gymnast. During World War I, he interned as a nurse and developed rehabilitation and strength equipment. In 1926, he and his wife opened their first pilates gym in New York City catering to dancers. Here he taught a combination of posture, breathing, and mat training using specially designed equipment. He emphasized grace and a flowing motion outward from a strong center. His clients shared testimonials that they felt leaner and taller. They claimed pilates helped them to develop long, sleek muscles.

Although there is no research to support the thought that pilates lengthens muscle and enhances growth, pilates advocates are adamant that they redistributed their weight to create a new shape to their bodies. Pilates aficionados assert that they develop long, slender thighs and calves, a strong back, a flat tummy and a high tushie (butt), along with an invigorated, energized, countenance.

Five different pieces of equipment are used to train almost every muscle in the body. The equipment includes the Barrel, Cadillac, Chair, Pedipull, and Reformer. Using these pieces of equipment, students are instructed to perform a high number of repetitions using low weights at very high levels of intensity and focus.

Women in particular are attracted to pilates. Compared to spinning and cardio-kick boxing, pilates can offer a quiet, contemplative alternative. The pilates method includes exercise strategies that train your back and abdominal muscles promoting perfect posture both in and out of the gym. Pilates teaches you a variety of breathing techniques and lets you experience what your "neutral spine" is supposed to feel like when it is optimally aligned.

Pilates focuses on your posture. When your back is out of alignment, you require more energy to move—like a car with square wheels. Pilates allows you to become aware of your posture and, in turn, provides you with:

▸ More powerful fulcrums for strength training
▸ Better positioning for flexibility.

When practicing pilates, grace and perfect body alignment are your goals. The balance, grace, and body control you gain during pilates can then transfer to your daily activities.

MIND/BODY COMBINATIONS. Above are mentioned only a few mind/body exercise regimes. When you create your own mind/body program, choose the activity that is right for you, and remember that you are not limited to a single mind/body strategy. Currently in the fitness industry, combinations of different activities are in vogue. For example, yoga combined with aerobics (a.k.a. yogaerobics) is one way to assimilate mind/body strategies. Another example is a combination of cardio-kickboxing and taijiquan.

A popular, less demanding mind/body combination is *chi-yoga*. This practice is aimed at teaching you to balance your mind, body, and spirit. Yoga relaxation strategies help decrease tension and stiffness in your body. Through chi-yoga you will improve your strength, flexibility, endurance, posture, and confidence as well as your breathing and concentration habits. If you plan to try chi-yoga be sure you choose a certified instructor. Specifically, look for an instructor who can help you monitor your postures according to your individual physical needs and goals. If you have a bad back, knees, or an injured rotator cuff, your instructor can help you work around your difficulty.

Research has shown that a relaxed focus has a profound effect on your physiology. Decreased blood pressure, heart rate, and sympathetic stress hormones are just a few of the moderating effects of mind/body training. Pre- and post-tests like the Profile of Mood States (POMS), Spielberger's State-Trait anxiety inventory, and the Cook Medley Hostility Scale verify dramatic psycho-physiological changes. Research aside, if you try a mind/body strategy and you expect to see positive results, chances are you will.

LESS TRADITIONAL MIND/BODY COMBINATIONS. We know that punching and kicking can improve your martial arts, and meditation can enhance your mindfulness. However, are martial arts and meditation mutually exclusive activities? Or do these strategies provide a cross-training benefit? That is, does one activity help the other? Benson's research, presented later in this book, suggests that repetitive physical activity can help you achieve the relaxation response, especially if you are mindful of each punching combination or other activity you may do in repetition.

The principle of specificity of training (belief that if you practice a particular skill, you expect improvement in *that* skill only) suggests that meditation may not improve your martial arts and vice versa. Another similar theory proposes that one will respond to the specific adaptation of an imposed demand (e.g., if you overload your muscles with weights, your muscles will grow stronger, but if you perform biceps curls for your arms, your legs will not get bigger). Such analogies support the supposition that martial arts may not improve your mindfulness. The fact is that this supposition could not be further from the truth.

Frankly, you should practice both physical and mindfulness training. Rather than physically training to reach a spiritual goal or meditating for hours in hopes of winning a martial arts championship, focus both your practice and training to reach your specific target.

That is not to say you cannot practice mindfulness to improve your martial arts performance, or physically train to improve your mindfulness. For example, while punching, focus on your punch. Allow your inhalation-exhalation cycle to coincide with each punch. If your mind drifts from your breathing, gently remind yourself to focus. After awhile, let your mind focus on your breath or nothing at all. Soon you will punch without thought. No thought means you are punching in the moment and nothing else occupies your mind. You are simply punching. This strategy will help you to achieve mindfulness.

We humans have grown accustomed to performing a variety of activities simultaneously. Listening to a Walkman while practicing *kata,* reading while watching television, or playing cards while listening to the radio are routine. It is more difficult to just do *kata,* just read, just play cards, or just focus on each punch or kick. This is mindful meditation, and after awhile, mindful meditation is an end in itself.

CHAPTER 2

Activation and Concentration

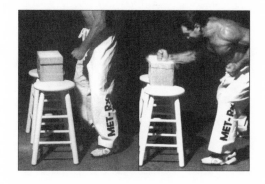

✳ Activation and Concentration ✳

Activation

Activation is the act of getting pumped up, psyched, and mentally prepared. It is synonymous with the sports psychology term arousal. Activation is not anxiety. Although anxiety involves increased arousal, anxiety arousal grows from worry and negative thoughts and feelings.

If you are too excited or bored, you will not perform your best. Having the jitters inhibits fine motor movement such as throwing triple consecutive kicks or putting a golf ball. However, if you are too relaxed, you will not perform well either. The key to peak performance is finding your optimum level of activation. You need to be mindful, depending on what you are doing and how well you are doing it, of symptoms of anxiety and boredom so that you can manipulate your activation level accordingly.

Generally a higher activation level leads to better performance, especially if you are confident with what you are doing. This is not true for everyone, however, so you must experiment to find the activation level that works for you. Mindfulness is the awareness that can help you do this. Mindfulness allows you the sensitivity to look at your activation level and determine if raising it or lowering it will help or hurt your performance. One way to mindfully monitor your activation is to rate your arousal on a scale from 1–10 where one is your lowest and ten is your highest. By doing so, you will know if you are too excited or too relaxed for your specific event. This can provide you with an objective measure to decide if you need to increase or decrease your activation.

TO INCREASE YOUR ACTIVATION:

- ▸ Be sure to warm up.
- ▸ Increase your breathing cadence.
- ▸ Focus on what you are doing instead of feeling tired.
- ▸ Listen to your favorite music.
- ▸ Imagine yourself as fast and powerful.
- ▸ Pretend you have a crowd watching and draw energy from it.

TO DECREASE YOUR ACTIVATION:

- ▸ Be mindful.
- ▸ Breathe slowly from your belly.
- ▸ Repeat calming words to yourself like "relax."
- ▸ Think about your performance, not on the outcome.
- ▸ Do not focus on whether or not you will win.
- ▸ Notice the difference between tension and relaxation in your entire body.
- ▸ Slow down, do not rush.

RELAXATION AND ACTIVATION

There are a variety of relaxation techniques that bring about a relaxation response. One of them is progressive relaxation. Progressive relaxation allows you to contract and relax muscle groups until you feel and understand the difference between tension and relaxation. During this process you first learn to contract and relax each muscle group separately, then with practice you can combine the groups so you relax your whole body at once. When you can do so, you will be able to relax at will. Reminding yourself to relax, however, is the hardest part. If you let things get out of your grasp, before you know it, you will be nervous and out of control. If you remember to remain mindful, relaxation is natural.

Below is an example of a progressive relaxation strategy:

RELAXATION STRATEGY

Mentally select various muscle groups within your body. Before you actually start, close your eyes and enjoy the rest for a minute or so. Accept any perceptions or emerging thoughts and let them pass by like leaves floating on a creek. Do not ponder or brood, and try not to daydream. If an important idea surfaces, return to it later when your exercise is finished. Begin contracting and relaxing the muscle groups in the order you selected. Tighten each group and hold the tension for about five seconds, and then relax for about thirty seconds. As you do this, focus your inner perception on the muscles that you have just exercised. You will sense that the process of relaxation will progress after you release the muscles. Let it happen that way and enjoy it. Repeat one time for each muscle group.

When you are finished, keep your eyes closed for a short while and enjoy the rest a little longer. Breathe in deeply, and move your fingers and toes playfully. Continue to breathe deeply and stretch yourself, and then open your eyes. This breathing and stretching makes sure that your circulation is reactivated. When you are finished you will feel quite refreshed.

Deep breathing enhances the effects of progressive relaxation. With each exhalation tension will release in your muscles; notice the difference between a tensed and relaxed state. Practice relaxation techniques according to your needs and goals. Personalize your mind/body strategies to fit your lifestyle.

Learning to relax may be the single most important lesson you can accomplish. You already know how to lie down on a cozy couch and watch television in a stupor, but this is not relaxation. The relaxation that I am talking about is recognizing your symptoms of anxiety and spontaneously allowing yourself to relax. This is mindfulness, and it requires practice. Sometimes we can have a difficult time understanding our own distresses and anxieties. It is very important for you to recognize these feelings so that you can identify the source of the problem and do something about it.

In the realm of anxiety-causing emotions, fear is paralyzing. Fearful thoughts snowball. For example, if your fear of martial arts competition is caused by anxiety about losing, your experiences reinforce your tendencies. However, if you are mindful of your fear, and enter one competition without fear of failure, you can open doors to an exciting future.

You can modify your thoughts to diminish anxiety and to relax. Your thoughts create your reality. Be mindful of them and, if necessary, change them. Mindfulness allows you to enjoy any situation. There is no one prescription or blueprint. Recognize your self-defeating talk and take an active stand. For example, if you decide you dislike travel, you will. If travel is something you really want to do, list the reasons you hesitate to travel and handle each problem one at a time. If you are compulsive about wasting time, invest in a laptop computer. Allow late departures and arrivals to teach you to be flexible. Plan ahead and make appropriate arrangements. Are you homesick? Make time to call or send email to your family often and spend quality time with them when you are home.

Anxiety and negativity surrounds us, so be mindful of anxious symptoms. Close your eyes and calm your thoughts. Breathe deeply, play with your pet, or hug your kids. Be mindful to remain relaxed during your fight with traffic or tournament competition. If you are mindful, you can handle any strife. There is nothing that can rattle you; your reactions are controlled, and you are prepared for anything. Your presence of mind will be inspiring to others, and people will recognize that you are different.

DECREASING ACTIVATION WITH MINDFULNESS

Many people frown from worry and guilt. They have lost their mindfulness or perhaps never found it. Their health has become overridden by excess. Take a trip to your local mall or department store and observe people shopping. Most are either harried or lethargic. Many are overweight. Activity and discipline are no longer the foundation of our culture. Only five percent of Americans eat right and exercise and less than ten percent are fit.

Those that do work out, pump iron to deafening music, cycle while talking on their cell phones or otherwise perform activities that distract them from their workouts. Mindfulness is a lost art. In our present culture, it seems more efficient to listen to a book on tape while jogging rather than attend to breathing or to practice *kata* to rock music rather than to focus on your imaginary opponent.

Practicing mindfulness is not hard or time consuming. It is simply a matter of focusing on what you are doing. When was the last time you watched a good movie? Was it so intense you were unconscious of your surroundings? Were you so engrossed you forgot you were hungry, thirsty, or needed to go to the restroom? When the movie ended, did you rush to the restroom? The object of your meditation was exemplary concentration. In this case your concentration was on the movie.

When you immerse yourself in martial arts, and let distractions in one ear and out the other, every act and thought is meditation. You can meditate anytime, anywhere, while waiting in line, riding in a car, or sitting quietly with your eyes closed. Meditation is mindfulness. It helps you to maintain your focus. Mindfulness allows you to focus your attention, concentrate on your studies, martial arts, or take part in social interactions. Mindfulness allows you to devote your attention to any movement, idea, or any project that is worthwhile.

Try staring at a photograph of a perfect side kick. Focus your attention for two minutes. Then close your eyes. Mindfully bring back the side kick. See it with your eyes closed. Let your visualization become your focus. This is a form of meditation. The object of your meditation can be prayer, music, or a bowl of cereal. It does not matter, just enjoy it.

Meditation is non-competitive. Do not start out by saying, "I must meditate for twenty minutes or I have failed." Rather, meditate for as long or as little as you want. The process is what is important, not the goal. Meditation is a skill, the same as practicing martial arts. Mindful meditation becomes easier with practice. The more you rehearse, the better you become. Do not worry if you are a slow learner. Concern about your progress will only impede your improvement.

For most people, it is difficult to deal with silence. Watching television, playing solitaire, or staring out the window is a lot easier than sitting meditation. Meditation requires discipline, and the benefits are enormous. Take a moment to close your eyes and focus on your breath. Say "relax" with each exhalation. Can you do this for five minutes? Probably. Can you do it for five minutes without a distraction? Probably not. The discipline required to meditate helps you to conquer yourself. Meditation improves your mindfulness, which carries over into every aspect of your life.

Delayed gratification, relaxation, and focus are the foundations of mindful meditation. Although mindful meditation is beneficial, it can also have profound effects on performance activation. Activation varies on a continuum from low (deep sleep) to high (extreme excitement). It involves both a physiological response (e.g., increased heart rate) and psychological process (e.g., appraisal of an event). High activation makes you alert and energizes you. The essence of meditation is focusing your attention. Mindful meditation brings back your focus when you are distracted and will have positive effects on your ability to control your activation.

The following is an exercise that you can use to practice mindful meditation.

STEP ONE

- ► Sit comfortably in a chair and close your eyes.

- ► Focus on one goal (e.g., spiritual, physical, psychological, emotional, social, or financial).

- ► See, feel, and experience yourself having reached your goal.

- ► See, feel, and experience all of the rewards of having reached your goal.

STEP TWO

- ► See yourself the way you are. Be objective.

- ► See yourself exactly as you would like to be.

- ► Take a moment to merge the way you are with the way you would like to be.

- ► Finally, see your new self as a combination of all of your best traits.

Take a moment to notice your physical state. Are you tense? Are your teeth clenched? Try to relax them. If it does not come to you at first, that is okay, do not try so hard.

RESEARCH ON MEDITATION

The original studies on the physiology of Transcendental Meditation were published in *Science, American Journal of Physiology,* and *Scientific American* in 1970 through 1972. These studies found that Transcendental Meditation (TM) produces a physiological state known as restful alertness. During this state it was shown that the body showed significant reductions in respiration, minute ventilation, tidal volume, and blood lactate, as well as increased basal skin resistance (which basically means you are more relaxed). At the same time, the body is alert rather than asleep, as indicated by an abundance of alpha brain waves. Dr. Keith Wallace concluded that restful alertness is a fourth state of consciousness. The other three states of consciousness include wakefulness, dreaming, and deep sleep.

Other research has shown that those who meditate were more relaxed outside of their meditative state as well. Baseline levels of respiration, heart rate, plasma lactate, and skin resistance were all lower. Medical researchers have found reduced risk of cardiovascular disease such as high blood pressure and high serum cholesterol.

Mindfulness

Your past affects your future, especially a painful past. Your future unconsciously hides from and combats a painful past. Reliving painful moments is very difficult, and we do whatever we can to avoid it. If it feels as if you are reliving a painful moment or experience, change the situation. Change begins with understanding where you are at a particular moment. This is mindfulness. When I broke the twenty-four-hour cycling record, I experienced pain the entire ride. I was never able to push myself to that level of pain again.

Thinking about the past may cause you regrets, and you may be nervous or fearful of your future. Do not dwell in the past or live in the future. These are habits. Bouncing from the past to the future is not living it is merely existing. Mindfulness is living in the present. I found myself repeatedly asking my children "What do you have going for tomorrow?" and "What did you do while I was gone last weekend?"

Inadvertently, I was teaching my kids to live for the future and relive their past. Now I ask, "Do you want to practice karate?" or "How are you feeling?" It is okay to learn from the past and plan for the future, but you do not have to relive the past or be anxious about the future over and over again.

If you live in the moment, you learn a lot about yourself. If you are mindfully engaged in your passion, you feel right. You are optimistic and courageous and in control. It is easy to punch and kick if you have purpose. You know yourself better than anyone; decide your own purpose. Your purpose:

YOUR PURPOSE...

- ▸ is chosen by you.

- ▸ must challenge you.

- ▸ must help you to grow.

- ▸ should be positive.

- ▸ should be beneficial to others.

When you first become aware of something, for an instant there is pure mindfulness. A few seconds later, you label it and conceptualize it. Mindfulness is usually that very short period of time that occurs just before you begin to analyze. Once you analyze a situation the mindfulness disappears. Right now you are mindful as you focus on these words. Once you realize that you are focusing the mindfulness disappears.

In my karate class, I teach my students to be mindful of their opponent. They are taught to focus on the solar plexus with a soft, vague awareness. They learn to see the rest of their opponents' bodies using peripheral vision. They are mindful of their opponents without any preconceived notions about what they will do. They are relaxed and not worried about their opponents' reactions. They are simply mindful.

Mindfulness reflects what presently happens and exactly the way it is happening. There is no past or present; there is no judgment. You simply observe without praise or criticism. You are never surprised or taken off balance because you have no preconceived notions. When you expect nothing you can handle anything. Mindfulness is the perception of what is. There is no fear, worry, or infatuation. There is no good or bad, and positive and negative are equally experienced.

Mindfulness requires no thought, only observation. Attention is all that matters. In a martial arts situation, there is no time for analysis. Mindfulness leads to an automatic reaction or you will lose. Mindfulness generally occurs before your thoughts. It is real-time. Mindfulness has no ego. Therefore, if you are mindful, there is no pain. That is not to say that you will not notice pain, you will but it will not be attached to you. You are simply an objective observer of the pain. (This is an advanced concept.)

Mindfulness is part of the process; it is not the product you try to achieve. If you are mindful, you are not worried about a goal; you are focusing on the task at hand. Please do not be misled: mindfulness is not cold and unfeeling. When you are mindful, you are excited and emotional, but you are always in control of those emotions.

When you are mindful of your breathing and inexplicably find yourself worrying about your dinner options, it is your mindfulness that gently pulls you back to your breath. It was not conscious thought, just a mindful reminder to focus on your breath. If you practice martial arts it is mindfulness that brings your attention back to your imaginary opponent.

To take a step forward, recognize your needs, but do not be controlled by them. Although to the rest of the world you are living normally, challenge yourself:

STRATEGIES FOR CHALLENGING YOURSELF

---

1. Expect nothing: Do not get distracted by your expectations about results.

2. Do not try too hard or force anything. Violence, aggression, exaggeration, or intent to achieve too much can lead to tension. Allow your effort to be steady.

3. Do not rush. Know that whatever you are doing will take as long as it takes. Settle in for the long haul. Anything valuable takes time.

4. Accept everything. Let come what comes. If good happens, fine. If bad things arise, that is okay too. Be comfortable with whatever happens. Do not fight with things you cannot change. Be mindful and go on.

5. Allow yourself to flow like water. Relax and stay focused. Remain mindful, noncompetitive, and activated.

6. Be kind to yourself. Plan on making mistakes, learn from them, and they will take you one step closer to your goal.

7. Learn from everything. Be flexible and experience as much as possible.

8. Do not think of obstacles as problems; rather, they are challenges. Remember you have no problems, only challenges. Look upon negatives as opportunities for experience.

9. Do not analyze. You do not need to know everything. Sometimes reasoning just gets in the way.

10. Do not be competitive. Simply improve on your skills. Whether you are better than another is a moot point.

There is a difference between awareness of a thought and thinking it. Awareness of your thought is mindfulness. Awareness of a thought requires distance between you and your thought. When you are emotionally tied to your thought, it draws you in and can take control of you. Conscious thought causes your heart to flutter and your muscles to contract. Be aware of these thoughts. If necessary, diminish their activation-producing effects.

Regular mindful practice allows you to become aware and allows you to let go of your unconscious desires and worries. Mindfulness is moment to moment. It is living fully in the present, and it allows you to accept whatever is happening whether you like it or not. Through mindful practice, you will live life to its fullest and experience every second—good or bad.

We all live in a flurry of change everyday. When you practice mindfulness regularly, you learn to accept change. No two moments in your life are ever the same. Being mindful allows you adapt to the normality of change. If you resist change, stress is bound to follow. Be mindful of each moment, one action at a time. The acceptance of change does not come naturally to most people. For unexplained reasons, people hold onto phobias and anxiety. Some are addicted to tension, choosing stress rather than consciously transforming inner conflict into peace of mind. Stress and continual change is not a bad thing. If you practice, you can cope with anything. Soon you will react to each moment with proper awareness and clarity. Anxiety and worry will not cloud your thinking, and stress diminishes because you simply respond to the present.

Practicing daily mindfulness is not easy. Yet, the benefits are immeasurable. Train yourself to focus on the here and now. Keep yourself balanced, centered, and peaceful no matter what. Become aware of the symptoms of anxiety, symptoms that normally blind you to what is really happening. Through the years you have developed patterned reactions to stresses. Be aware that these reactions can make it difficult for you to be mindful. Your previous experiences influence your perception of the present, so you are unconsciously controlled by past fears and worries. This creates undesirable reactions. Unconsciously, you allow past experiences to control your present. This attachment to the past can be broken with mindfulness.

When past feelings and thoughts control you, mindfulness disappears, and you manifest uncontrolled worry. Worry overloads your present thought patterns, is a waste of your time, and creates anxiety. By unconsciously creating a worst case scenario, your body tries to fight-or-flight. The adrenal overload that occurs during this response is exhausting, especially if you do this day after day. Such stress can cause headaches, backaches, high blood pressure, and heart arrhythmia. Worry snowballs, and before you know it you are out of control.

Become aware of how you handle anxiety and fear. Look at yourself objectively so you have a starting point. Practice mindfulness regularly to let go of unconscious worries. Know you can handle anything if you give yourself the chance. Signs of successful mindfulness include decreased: fear, impatience, vengeance, confusion, and guilt. These are replaced with love, patience, compassion, clarity, and wisdom. These transformations, however, do not occur overnight. They take practice.

Mindfulness is simply becoming aware of what you are doing right now. Take a moment for yourself and try this: Assume a comfortable sitting position. Breathe. Become aware of your breath and focus on your breathing. Just inhale and exhale. Be a part of each breath. If you notice a distraction, say, "that is okay," and come back to your breath. Let nothing else bother or disturb you. Simply inhale, exhale, and focus. At first you may find breath-focus difficult, much like when your parents told you to sit still. With practice, however, breath-focus will be relaxing and you will feel balanced and secure.

Practice breathing five minutes a day. Add one minute a week until you are practicing for ten minutes.

Become an observer of your thoughts instead of becoming overwhelmed by them. This way, you handle your thoughts without mindlessly reacting to them. See your thoughts for what they are and focus on their meaning without negativity. This helps you understand your motivations.

A difficult aspect of mindfulness is being nonjudgmental. Become a silent witness of your thoughts and feelings. Almost like a documentary, just look for the facts without adding color to the story. This does not mean giving up and accepting hardship. Instead mindfully see the big picture and make plans to develop a conscious, clear plan of attack.

Deepak Chopra said, "You are the thinker behind the thought, the observer behind the observation, the flow of attention, the flow of awareness, the unbounded ocean of consciousness. When you have that on the experiential level, you spontaneously realize that you have choices, and that you can exercise these choices, not through some sheer will power but spontaneously." Dr. Chopra is talking about mindfulness.

MINDFULNESS REQUIRES QUIET TIME

Americans are physically, socially, and mentally stimulated almost all of the time. It is increasingly more and more difficult to find time to be alone. Lunch hours have turned into catch-up time and midmorning breaks are nonexistent. Cellular phones, pagers, and fax machines are a bane. Information provides tools to improve your life, and networking enhances your communication. You do, however, need time and privacy to figure it all out. You need to give yourself time to gain a mindful perspective.

It has been found that after experiencing an hour in a sensory deprivation tank, people experienced lower blood pressure, improved creativity, a more positive outlook, and higher mental functions. You need quiet time. Solitude allows you to mindfully organize and plan your day. We all do not have the opportunity to experience a sensory deprivation tank, but the good news is to experience mindfulness you do not need one. Just sit down alone and be by yourself. Uninterrupted minutes allow you to readjust, order your priorities and pay attention to your needs. Solitude provides rest and delivers energy unimagined.

Creative youngsters instinctively cherish their time alone. My eight-year-old son spends several hours a week interacting with imaginary martial arts characters. His little hands punch, kick, spin, and fly. At first, I thought this was peculiar. Now I understand that personal moments are a vital ingredient to enhanced creativity, mindfulness, and improved concentration.

Being alone does not mean you are lonely. Society sometimes labels people as antisocial if they prefer solitude and are seen unaccompanied. In our society eating lunch in the corner of a crowded cafeteria can be demoralizing. Yet it does not have to be. It depends on your attitude. Be mindful of your meal and enjoy it. Make time alone for yourself. Close the door to your office and perform taijiquan, meditate, or pray. In Japan there are places set aside specifically for people to be mindful and solitary.

Some people ultimately say no to crowded offices and harried lifestyles. For sanity's sake, they give up lucrative careers to pursue self-employment or a mindful profession. Not all of us can handle these extreme measures, but a few moments of quiet contemplation can do wonders. Those who meditate focus their *qi*, Zen masters contemplate *koans,* Thoreau walked around Walden Pond. Find what is good for you, and relax and focus.

Use solitary moments to enhance your mindfulness. Value personal time to discover who you are. Become sensitive to your thoughts, actions, and behaviors.

After a hard day, when you open your front door, instead of being barraged by information overload, sit down, relax, and prioritize. Let the answering machine pick up phone messages. There is no phone call more important than the tranquility you will gain through mindful meditation. Pamper yourself, listen to music, meditate, or pray. Mindful moments are their own end. Get in touch; mindfulness is there for the taking.

MINDFULNESS AND PAIN

Be sensitive to aches and pains that can become injuries or a sore throat that turns into a serious infection. Let your body provide your brain with the information required to maintain your training.

Enjoy the process more than the end result. We have all seen the thrill of victorious athletes broken but triumphant. Similarly, at one time or another we have all experienced defeat, even if the defeat was to a more experienced opponent. If circumstances control your happiness, you will rarely find joy. Be mindful of your emotions, and you will remain balanced.

LISTENING TO YOUR BODY

Mind/body strategies enhance your mindfulness, physical performance, and rehabilitation. Yet if your mind/body program is uncomfortable or if a so-called guru is telling you to do something that is not within your belief system, maybe it is not the right time or place to pursue that particular activity.

You may have become carried away with your martial arts and developed overtraining injuries. Pain and dysfunction are fraught with muscle tension and negative images. By allowing your mind to create an enhanced healing environment, healing an injury can be facilitated. Remaining relaxed keep your muscles from contracting. Use imagery to send blood to your injury to enhance your healing.

Control your emotional responses to pain (e.g., fight-or-flight response, anger, anxiety). Although Western medicine may not address mind/body techniques, most physicians will agree that stress exacerbates many disease processes. Go right to the source of your problem. Rehabilitation occurs under the best conditions. Relax and be mindful of your healing.

There is a link between relaxation and injury prevention since injuries are more likely to occur when there is tension in your muscles. When practicing your martial arts, it is imperative for you to be relaxed to experience peak performance. Become mindful of every move you make. By allowing yourself to become part of every strike and block, relaxation will become a welcome by-product.

Visualize your pain diminishing and you will heal. Use positive self-talk about your ability to cope with pain. Befriend your pain and let it help you to improve. Pushing too hard can cause you to re-injure yourself, but fearing pain may lead to an approach that may be too passive.

If pain stops you from performing your martial art, maintain your sense of identity and importance through other activities that help you feel good about yourself. Work around your pain or injury by being aware of your current level of function, then go beyond those limitations and imagine your future with an improved level of function.

Surround yourself with supportive people. Be creative, humorous, and positive in your approach to the daily inconveniences caused by your pain. Techniques such as progressive relaxation, breathing, and visualization can help to alleviate your pain. The best method to handle pain, however, is to develop an ongoing sense of mindfulness.

Your mind and body need to feel the difference between tension and relaxation. Starting with your feet and working up, alternate contracting your muscles, then relaxing them. Memorize the feeling of relaxation. Relax whenever possible to combat pain and be mindful of how you are feeling at all times.

Breath control helps you to modify your response to pain by focusing on your breath instead of your pain. When you experience pain, breathe freely and remain relaxed. Let your lungs fill completely by extending your diaphragm as you inhale, and feel the air move in and out of the bottom of your lungs. Release negative thoughts as you exhale. Mindful breathing allows you to focus on only your desires.

Imagery can provide you with a nurturing and healing environment. Use breathing and music to prepare. Then relax. Concentrate on total body wellness. Visualize a warm healing sensation moving cell by cell through your entire body. Focus on a painful area and imagine a cool, blue light massaging your pain away. Say to yourself, "I am healing, I am relaxed, my pain will disappear." Mindfulness is total objectivity about your pain.

Management of anxiety is also a form of pain management. Anxiety is invisible, but it is there. When you finally notice you are anxious, it may be too late. Be mindful of your initial symptoms of duress (stress with negative effects) so you can reverse your response immediately.

Some people perform unconscious repetitive activities to combat anxiety. Chewing your fingernails, toe tapping, and pencil thumping may be your way to combat anxiety. Herbert Benson, M.D., suggests better methods including walking, pedaling, or meditating. As a martial artist you can throw repetitive punches, kicks, strikes, and blocks. According to Benson, these monotonous activities relax your body and stop the production of stress hormones.

You might assume that developing the ability to relax and focus is sheer serendipity—that is, some people are fortunate enough to do so;

others cannot. Yet you also believe that for you it is different. Highs are short-lived and the doldrums never end. Be mindful of two concepts for peak performance: activation and focused concentration.

PROGRAMMING TO HANDLE PAIN

It is easy to take the middle of the road or walk the fence. I can punch and kick for hours at a steady state below my anaerobic threshold. Yet, when I speed, I huff and puff, and soon I quit. To reach optimum performance in any endeavor, learn to tolerate discomfort. Pushing beyond your anaerobic threshold is painful, and no one enjoys pain.

There are tricks, however, to making discomfort bearable. First, prepare. If your dentist activates his drill to bore a hole through your molar, you quickly become prepared to deal with the pain. Think for a moment how you do this. Either put yourself in another place, or mindfully prepare for the pain and welcome it. I prefer the latter. When I hear the whir of his drill, I say, "Welcome pain! Pain makes me stronger. The more pain I can endure now, the more pain I can handle later. There is no worthwhile goal that can be achieved without pain."

Daily pain associated with training seems to be a prerequisite for stunning performances. Sometimes it takes years of tedious, boring practice sessions. Olympic Taekwondo champions train day after day with little stimulation. Martial arts masters mindfully practice their art week after week perfecting their routines. Most successful competitors train year-round.

Acute physical pain, though, sometimes precedes prolific achievements. I watched a Taiwanese martial artist place his dislocated arm into his uniform so he could continue fighting. During another fight an American fighter clashed shins with a Korean; both fractured their tibias, yet both finished the fight. A former Olympian once admonished, "Winners are those who can hold their hands in the fire the longest." World record distance runner, Steve Prefontaine said, "I may be beaten, but you will have to bleed to do it." To be the best, martial artists give everything, sometimes with little reward. Most realize they have only one shot, and to make it, they must invest themselves fully. Many who are not associated with competition have difficulty comprehending the intensity of elite martial arts athletes. Olympic athletes have goals, not just dreams. If they just had dreams they would wake up every morning and wish they had gold medals hanging from their necks. Goals require action. Action requires mindfulness, especially if the object of your training is not realized.

Concentration and Focus

You are constantly bombarded by an endless array of internal and external stimuli. These include thoughts, emotions, and people trying to tell you what to do. With all of these distractions, it is difficult to focus. Be mindful of what is important, and discard the irrelevant. Selectively attend to relevant stimuli. Let the rest go in one ear and out the other.

Focus your undistracted attention for an extended period. Although this might seem arduous, it is not. Real focus is effortless. Some call it "the zone," "flow," or "being absorbed in the present" What makes focus a challenge is that your mind tends to shift to new stimuli. This was a survival instinct because your ancestors had to keep one eye open for an attack at all times. Learn to control your focus and hone your concentration like a laser. Here are some ways to improve your focus:

STRATEGIES TO IMPROVE FOCUS

- Change negative feelings and thoughts that distract you from your goals.

- Stay in the present. If something goes wrong, note it, and then adjust.

- Remind yourself to stay focused by using key words such as "relax, focus."

- Be process-oriented. If you are worried about succeeding, you probably will not.

- Add a ritual or consistent routine to your regimen. This will keep you grounded.

- When you are tired, be especially vigilant to minimize lapses in concentration.

- Focus and activation are very important. Be careful of over- or under-activation.

Imagine taking your dog for a walk. You hold tightly to the leash as you spot a cat in the distance. While holding the leash, let your dog go for it! Watch its motivation level! Observe how focused your dog is. This is pure unadulterated concentration. It may be for just a brief moment, but it is intense and true. Your dog has a will to achieve its goal at all costs. Although your dog did not set a long-term goal, its focus was all-encompassing. Let us not forget the other end of your dog's pursuit either, the cat. I am sure that cat did not just stand there and let you and Fido run at it at full gallop. The cat reacted instinctively to get out of there either by running away or by taking a ninety-degree turn up a tree. Animals, if we pay attention to their movements, can be wonderful inspirations to greater levels of concentration. You are much more intelligent than your dog. Try to attain its single-minded focus.

FOCUS AND YOUR WORKOUT

There are two components to your martial arts workout. The first and most obvious is the physical. The second is the influence that mindfulness has on your training and performance. Many instructors and coaches dismiss mindfulness. Yet it is through your ability to focus that peak performance is attained.

Just as your martial arts goal may be to train at a certain pace, to improve on your previous performance or to get fit, you should have mindfulness goals as well. The primary mind/body goal is to attain the highest level of appreciation for whatever you are doing. I consider it a privilege to train in the martial arts and I love every minute of my training. As you train, be mindful of your body's hormonal response. Your body responds to stress by secreting the sympathetic hormones epinephrine and norepinephrine, which are the fight-or-flight hormones. The fight-or-flight response masks fatigue and promotes feelings of well-being and euphoria. It will make you feel as if you can kick and punch forever. Be careful though, this is a physiological response. Too much enjoyment of this feeling can lead to overtraining.

VISUALIZATION AND IMAGERY ENHANCE
YOUR MARTIAL ARTS WORKOUT

Visualization is something you can practice anytime, anywhere, whether you are stuck on the runway or are on your way to your event. Mindful visualization is a concrete way to change your life. Your mind programs your body for peak performance. Your brain sends impulses down neuromuscular pathways to speed or slow your kicks. Visualize yourself as an achiever. Do not worry yourself into your next self-fulfilling prophecy. Take command over your thoughts and focus on a promising future. There is never a moment where you cannot create a momentous change. Use your mind during your free moments to create what you desire. Whether you decide to view yourself as a ravenous eating machine or a mindful martial artist, the choice is yours.

As a youth, I wanted to be good at something but I could not find a talent. My fingers were too slow to be a lead guitarist and my serve was too weak to play professional tennis. After I passed my black belt test, one of the judges approached me and said, "After watching your *katas* I thought you were too mechanical, but having seen you fight, if you ate, slept, and drank karate you could be a champion." His words inspired me to my greatest efforts. I was able to maintain motivation through drudgery and pain of struggling. I used imagery to improve my concentration to "see" myself sparring prior to my actual event. I made my goals as specific and detailed as possible and structured them so they were attainable.

The images you create are powerful, and they can change your reality. Beware, though, that these images can spur you to greatness or hold you back. Your visualizations are your choice. By visualizing your mission and the benefits of your martial art and by moving toward your goal, you can increase you activation. Pretend to be focused or waste time worrying about losing. The choice is yours. If you are mindful, you will always make the correct choice.

You can use internal or external imagery to sharpen your focus. Imagery is a mental technique that programs your mind to respond by using your senses to create or recreate an experience. When you imagine yourself performing martial arts, you are using imagery. Imagery helps you rehearse new kicks, practice existing moves, and prepare for an event. Studies show that imagery lowers your anxiety and increases your self-confidence. Because you are totally objective in your imagery, it is truly a mindful experience.

Imagery, like mindfulness, improves with practice. Imagery is something that you can lie down and practice for an entire thirty minutes, few minutes or even seconds. If you have difficulty performing imagery try the following:

STRATEGIES FOR IMAGERY PRACTICE

- Think in pictures.
- Look at photos or videos prior to using imagery to stimulate your practice of imaging.
- Remain in a quiet, relaxed, and calm environment.
- Make the imagery seem as realistic as possible by including all of your senses.
- Visualize in full color and detail. Let your emotions become involved.
- Practice imagery regularly as it is a skill that improves with practice.
- Believe that imagery works, because the placebo effect (if you think it works, it will) is quite powerful.
- Stay relaxed and focused when practicing imagery.
- Internal imagery is most effective. Picture yourself performing from your own perspective, rather than viewing yourself as if watching television.
- Only imagine yourself performing well. This will boost your confidence and improve your performance.

See and feel yourself achieving your martial arts goals. Your mind's eye is a tool to bolster your confidence and jazz up your performance. Practice mindfulness every chance you get. Mindfulness is kind of like a referee; it will help you to make proper decisions about where to focus. For example, if you find yourself waiting in line, do not agonize over it; use that time to relax and concentrate on your goal. Enjoy a sense of productivity, and use these moments to truly focus.

When you perform imagery, use your senses: be sure to see, hear, feel, smell, and taste. The image you create is a mindful representation of what you have experienced or what you hope to experience. Imagery also helps you to code, store, and express information. Every time you daydream, dream, reminisce, or plan, you use imagery. Imagery is a right-brain creative strategy. It is much more than just sitting in a rocking chair visualizing bygone days.

Imagery also affects your immune system and your muscle and organ function. Tap your foot on the floor, then explain how you did that. Scientists cannot explain how you can tell yourself to tap your foot and then do it. Now, speed your heart rate. That is more difficult. You cannot just say, "okay, heart rate, speed up." Imagine for a moment, however, that you just won the lottery, and you will automatically experience tachycardia!

Imagery and visualization are powerful tools. Imagery of relaxing or exciting scenes can affect your heart rate, blood pressure, respiratory patterns, oxygen consumption, carbon dioxide elimination, brain wave rhythms and patterns, electrical characteristics of your skin, local blood flow, temperature, gastrointestinal motility, secretions, hormone levels and immune system function. Imagery helps you to relax and be comfortable in any situation as well as increase or decrease your activation levels. Imagery lets you modify, reduce, or eliminate discomfort. Imagery is your bridge to creativity. Use it every chance you get.

REACHING THE NEXT LEVEL

Be objective. Practice mindfulness. Imagine your goal. See yourself as having achieved it. Describe how reaching your goal will help others. Visualization is a great tool for success. The following are some things that may curtail your efforts to reach your potential. If you are aware of them then you can do something about it.

PITFALLS

- ► fear of failure

- ► fear of success

- ► fear of commitment

▸ fear of change

▸ fear of cost

To succeed you must believe that you deserve whatever it is that you want. Whether it is a little or a lot, you must visualize that you have gotten everything you believed you should. Imagine your life as a house that you have outgrown. It is time to add a new wing. Do not let guilt get in the way. You are not selfish or asking too much. It is simply the time to move to the next level.

To realize the next level, make a change, but change because you choose to do so. Do not be a victim of circumstance. When you decide to change, remember that success and failure come from the same effort. It is your effort that matters. If you fail, simply alter your course. Mistakes and failures are teaching tools that point you in the right direction. Both success and failure are your motivation.

When mistakes are overwhelming, step back and regain your composure. Remove yourself from the situation, calm down, and relax. Ease back from your racing heart and quick judgments so that you can find your center. Make realistic decisions concerning what you can do and visualize how to be different. Advance yourself a little at a time. Reward yourself for reaching a meaningful turning point and reward yourself for completing your goal. Most importantly, reward yourself for your diligence. Be open to surprises, the unexpected, new experiences, other points of view, and your inner voice.

Every problem you encounter has the possibility to do one of the following:

1. Become a solution.
2. Go away.
3. Change.

Recall the last six months of your life and make note of changes that you have made. Everything in your life is born in your mind. The more you focus on something, the more you become it. You have achieved success before and you will continue to be successful. Be mindful of your thoughts. Your thoughts are your possessions. They are your truth. Your thoughts are the basis for everything you say and do. Changing your thoughts changes your actions. That which matters is not what happens to you, it is what happens inside you. This simple fact affords you complete control over your life. Your reality is based on what you think, not what happens or what others try to make you believe. The thoughts you have affect your future.

Find your strengths and focus on them. Your strengths are those things in which you are confident; they are effortless for you. Strengths are what propel you over the top and provide you with limitless energy.

Although you should focus on your strengths, be sure to acknowledge your weaknesses. Your weaknesses haunt your thoughts and question your confidence. After I perform *kata* I may receive nine favorable scores and one that is unfavorable. Guess on which one my attention focuses? If you think you are good, others will also think you are good. If you blame yourself, others will blame you. If you trust yourself, others trust you.

Although you visualize yourself achieving goals, be careful of your expectations. Picture the best, but expect nothing. Your visualizations and imaging should not be misconstrued as process equals product. Instead, be prepared for any reality. If you believe all of your visualizations will manifest, then you will be disappointed. Mentally rehearse all for which you hope, but be completely content with wherever you are. That way there are no expectations and no disappointments. When your visualization comes true, enjoy the surprise of it all.

A forty-eight-year-old man signed up for my martial arts class. He had not worked out in twenty years, but he envisioned himself doing the Chinese splits as he had in his youth. Within weeks of beginning my class, he could nearly execute a Chinese split. Similarly, an Olympic gold medallist gushed upon winning, "You can do it. If you stick with it long enough, your dreams will come true." Spend a few minutes just before sleep mentally preparing for your training session. Visualize yourself enjoying your workout. Feel energy surging through your body. "See" a perfect model of your form. Feel yourself as fast and powerful. Relish the concept of moving toward your ideal self. Mindfulness brings your real self and your ideal self closer together.

Integration = Activation + Concentration

Integration is a term I coined to sum up all of the feelings and attitudes associated with peak performance. Integration is different for all of us. Some common results of integration include feeling relaxed and focus, jazzed, pumped up, in the zone, ready, alert, and mindful. Integration feels right. When you are in it, you know it is the place to be. When you are out of it, you want to climb back in. Once you understand the characteristics of integration, the easier it will be to relive it.

When you are mindful, integration will follow. Whether you are waiting in line, watching television, or arguing with your spouse, you can be integrated. Integration requires a constant state of mindfulness and a continuous sense of self-reflection. Once you know the rules you can summon integration at will. It is a conscious feeling that can be reached by everyone. Most of us are content to hang our heads in day-to-day drudgery, but you do not have to if you just realize that all it takes is a second or two every hour to become mindfully integrated.

The following checklist can help you to achieve integration anytime, anywhere:

STRATEGIES FOR ACHIEVING INTEGRATION

---

1. Regulate your activation level. You should strive to be never too excited, too bored, or too tired.

2. Use your sense of humor in every situation.

3. Keep your mind on your individual focus of attention.

4. Use your emotions to help you pump up or relax.

5. Have a sense of kinesthetic balance. That is wherever you are, whatever you are doing, remain in control.

6. Be strong. Know that your body can handle any physical effort.

7. Be flexible. Understand that things may not go as planned. Handle any glitches or emergencies with control.

8. Handle success and failure the same. Overreaction is not an option.

9. Cope with physical and emotional pain.

10. Increase perseverance and tenacity with practice.

11. Be confident. You are a functioning human being, no better or worse than anyone.

———————————————————

Variables Affecting Mindfulness

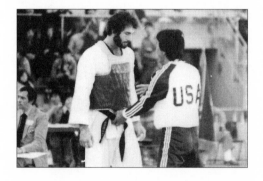

✳ Variables Affecting Mindfulness ✳

Self-Esteem

In our society a lot of effort has been put into the feel-good generation. The media capitalizes all the time on the need to increase our self-esteem. It is important to note, however, that self-esteem simply means how good you feel about yourself, regardless of whether or not your feelings have any basis in reality. For example, criminals including murderers and rapists, have demonstrated high levels of self-esteem especially during the crimes they commit.

Because self-esteem is not necessarily based in reality, it may not necessarily be true that you need more self-esteem. What you probably need to do is to boost your confidence. Confidence is how you feel about yourself based on what you have accomplished. By understanding the meanings of self-esteem and confidence you can see that there is a huge difference between your perception of your worth versus your worth based on your achievements. Remaining mindful about your accomplishments keeps you grounded.

I am not saying that to become a martial arts master all you need to do is feel good and be confident. What I am suggesting is that you need to look at your direction and goals and come up with a feeling about yourself based on where you are and where you would like to be. By doing so, you will not waste time trying to reach a level that may be unachievable to you at the present moment.

If you manufacture a high level of self-esteem based on zero reality, your house of cards will eventually crumble. To make progress, be confident in your accomplishments and have the foresight to set goals that are within your grasp. Then, day-by-day, mindfully achieve short- and long-term goals one at a time. Your goal-orientated mindfulness will allow you to be in the moment and not rely on insidious expectations for success.

Confidence

Confidence is a combination of your thoughts, feelings, and actions. Confidence provides you with a belief and is usually related to enhanced martial arts performance. Although it seems as if only the great ones have confidence, confidence can be improved; you just have to work at it.

To be confident, be sure your thoughts are process-oriented. Do not let the notion of failure enter your mind. Believe in your abilities and do not become discouraged or threatened. Pay attention to your body language because confidence will show here. When you achieve your goals—and you will achieve them—do not let success overwhelm you. It is easy to be confident if you are truly mindful of the difference between success and failure, but confidence without competence is a fragile situation. If you are overconfident and have no applicable skills and experience, you will not easily succeed. For success you need skill, practice, and experience. Confidence is just the icing on the cake that makes everything go just the way you planned.

Although confidence and success go hand in hand, remember you do not always have to succeed to be confident. Yet if you are not confident, you will probably not be successful. If you believe in yourself mindfully, self-doubt and anxiety cannot distract you. Confidence and mindfulness go hand in hand. Practice of mindfulness will ground you so that you will not appear arrogant.

The following are helpful strategies that will help improve your confidence.

STRATEGIES FOR IMPROVING YOUR CONFIDENCE

- ► Increase your personal fitness. It will improve your martial arts performance ability and your self-image.

► Once a week remind yourself of your strengths.

► Replace negative thoughts with positive affirmations such as "I can do it."

► Act confident, even when you are not.

► Improve your weaknesses until they become your strengths.

Motivation

Are you motivated to succeed or just to avoid failure? Successful mindful motivation is positive, goal-oriented, and anxiety reducing. Enjoy each day and, rather than accept what comes your way, relish each moment as a step closer to your goals. There is no doubt that a mindful approach is the best way to live.

There is a beauty in mindfulness that lies in the journey not just the result. By being directed toward a single, moment-to-moment goal, all distractions are removed from the equation. Have fun with the process more than the achievement, and savor each tiny victory along the way. Remember not to dwell on these tiny victories, though, because to do so is to live in the past and not in the moment.

Try these techniques to improve your motivation to success.

STRATEGIES FOR MOTIVATION

► Look forward to the thrill of competition but remain relaxed and focused.

► Do not hold yourself back. Your mindfulness will keep you balanced. Go for it no matter what.

Goal Setting

Goal setting is a powerful motivational tool. Setting both short- and long-term goals helps direct you toward improved martial arts performance by mindfully attaining your goals. Goals let you progress beyond fears that may be preventing you from being your best, and they allow you to be in control of what you do in your life. If you remain mindful of your goals, you will handle your successes and failures equally.

To maximize your goal-setting ability and subsequent performance, aim for improving your skills. As explained further in this text, if you mindfully set your goals, you will be process-oriented and display more intrinsic motivation, produce more effort, and possess greater endurance than those who just want to win. Do not define your performance level based on your competition. Choose to block, kick, or punch as fast and as powerfully as you can. If you have no concern for the outcome, winning will take care of itself.

If you are mindful, setting goals will improve your martial arts performance as well as your practice sessions. Your expectations will be realistic, and you will be challenged by new martial arts skills. As you develop these new tactics, your self-confidence will improve. Your pride will not be based on whether you win or lose. Your concentration will improve because you will have no concern of outcomes.

Here is how to do it:

STRATEGIES FOR GOAL SETTING

- ► Set measurable short- and long-term goals with target completion dates.
- ► Make sure your goals are challenging yet attainable.
- ► Keep in mind that your goals are performance-related and are not based on winning or losing.
- ► Adjust your goals when necessary.
- ► Set practice and performance goals.

Time Management

During my competitive years in ultra-cycling, I learned to make the best use of every moment. Time off of the bike meant losing ground to my competitors in the Race Across America (RAAM) and other competitive events. So as not to lose ground, I learned to eat on my bike, take a few winks of shut-eye, and even relieve myself without missing a pedal stroke. I trained six hours a day for this event, so my time off the bike had to be consolidated. I ate breakfast on the run, read mail during lunch, and answered emails while watching re-runs on TV.

Training on "RAAM TIME" was certainly not practicing mindfulness.

At the time I thought all of this was a pretty good trick. Doing two things at once seemed to be a huge time-saver. What I did not realize was that my heart was racing all the time. Even after my competitive years, I continued to live on "RAAM TIME." Whenever I could, I combined two or three activities to save time. I played with my kids while listening to a television program. I pedaled a stationary bike while typing on my computer. Life was good, or at least I thought it was.

The trip to my physician and subsequent atrial fibrillation diagnosis was a wake-up call. Since my emergency room debut, I set new priorities. Worrying about my presentations was getting me nowhere fast. I realized that being a little late or keeping someone waiting a few minutes was okay. I needed to learn to curb my compulsions and to make each day more enjoyable. I no longer think so much about tomorrow. I know that each moment is a treat and mindfulness is a must.

Your work ethic, like mine, can drive you to distraction. Make play a priority and know that having fun is okay. Spend at least an hour a day having fun. Have a sense of humor and a desire to enjoy life. If you have children, they will show you how. If you do not have children, remember how it felt to be a child. Where is your imagination? What happened to games like chase, checkers, and chess?

There is no such thing as wasting time. If you practice mindfulness every moment can be productive, fruitful, or fun. It is up to you. Meditate to re-energize, enjoy quiet contemplation, or create a fantasy. While shadowboxing or driving your car, your thoughts can stir you more than any motion picture. When you finally spend time with your family, you can exist in the moment and enjoy it.

Time management is fine, but maintain your priorities as well. It is very easy to fall into believing that since you planned every moment, you are doing the right thing. Every choice you make should fall in line with your mission, goals, and ideals. Each day, perform a self-evaluation. Ask yourself, "Was I mindful?" Be sure you are on course. If not, re-evaluate and move on.

DAILY SELF-EVALUATION

- ▸ Focus on results not just on being busy.

- ▸ Do what is important, give up the rest.

- ▸ Use your time most effectively.
- ▸ Control distractions.
- ▸ Increase your effectiveness.
- ▸ Reduce stress.
- ▸ Be in control of what you do.
- ▸ Be productive and secure.
- ▸ Enjoy what you do.
- ▸ Give yourself quality time to relax *after* work.
- ▸ Plan.
- ▸ Get off of the adrenaline buzz of finishing in the nick of time.

Irrational Thinking

I associated worry with success. Worry was the magic bullet to speed me through traffic jams. If I remained calm and relaxed, traffic would not let up, or so I thought. From early on I became conditioned so that I associated worry and heartache with achievement. It seemed that in order to achieve my goals suffering was required. I thought shallow breathing, and unrestricted anxiety actually helped me achieve my goals as a matter of association, not through cause and effect. Becoming mindful changed my conditioned nature.

During a tennis match, I noticed that I hit better when I assumed I would miss the shot and if I was confident that I would blast a great return, I did not. I played my best when I assumed that I had no chance to win. After a few years of losing tennis matches, I realized there was a logical reason I performed better when I gave up. By giving up I created a no-pressure match. When I was supposed to lose, I played my best. If the match got tight, and I thought, "I could win," I would choke. I now understand that I created or relieved the pressure that affected my performance, not my opponent.

In karate tournaments my mindset was different. If I was not in the moment, I would get hit. Fighting in the ring taught me that worry, fear, and a negative attitude do not improve your performance.

Negativity is demoralizing. When negative thoughts trickle in from time to time, discard them. Rather than becoming paralyzed, transform negative vibes into positive energy to power your attack. Mindfulness changes your adrenaline overload into focused, powerful energy that allows you to achieve your best performance.

You can train yourself to change negative into positive. Stay mindful of the bright side. If something bad happens, know that it is transitory and that things will be good again. Have a sense of humor about everything, do not be afraid to laugh at yourself. Always choose a positive outlook. Utilize self-talk. Talking to yourself is a powerful tool. Talking to yourself in a positive way will help you reap the benefits. Take note of the suggestions that follow, they can help.

ACCENTUATE THE POSITIVE

Positive:

- ► Start recording your self-talk before, during, and after major events.

- ► Use imagery to remember how you have reacted in past situations.

- ► Decide that you are ready to change your negative talk to positive.

- ► Change a negative thought to a positive one immediately before it snowballs.

Cognitive distortions are internal messages you give yourself that sabotage your performance and your enjoyment. Such distractions can become automatic and you may not be aware of them. They are harsh, critical, and self-defeating. Mindfully replace your negative thoughts with positive affirmations. Below are some typical examples of cognitive distortions to avoid:

ELIMINATE THE NEGATIVE

Negative:

- ► All or Nothing. You did terrible. You could not find anything good about your martial arts performance. Although you may have won your age group and performed a personal best you feel you are a failure because you did not win the overall competition.

- ► Overgeneralization. You think, "If it happened once, it will happen again and again. For example, when a flight of mine was cancelled, I became gunshy of my next flight. I would think, "Will the next one be cancelled too? Would I be left stranded again?" It is very easy to fall into a trap of associating experiences that are painful.

Become mindful of your self-talk. Replace all-or-nothing attitudes and overgeneralizations with positive thoughts, feelings, and affirmations.

How you mentally instruct yourself can either hurt or help you. Learn to make simple adjustments in your self-talk to improve your performance and always remain positive. Similarly, when you are in your doctor's office, tell him or her how you want to feel, rather than barraging the doctor with how bad you feel. Use a positively framed strategy and request what you want your doctor to do for you. By mentally ordering what you want, you are more apt to achieve your desired outcomes.

Fear

Fear is a negative emotion brought about by real or imagined danger or evil. In martial arts situations, fear is caused by thoughts of making a mistake, appearing incompetent, or losing. Fear leads to a state of high arousal, impaired focus, indecision, loss of confidence, and contracted muscles. Fear helped our primitive ancestors increase their adrenaline to fight off wild beasts and survive. However, in society today, fears snowball into greater fears tomorrow. Fear makes your anticipated event seem even worse, causing you to become careful and tentative. In martial arts competition, this phenomena is referred to as "The Choke." The enemy of fear is mindfulness. Since fear is generated in your mind, mindfulness squelches it.

STRATEGIES FOR HANDLING FEAR

- ▸ Do not worry about what others think of you. What you think is what really matters.

- ▸ Think like a winner all of the time. Imagine what it would be like to reach your goals.

- ▸ Visualize your winning moments and forget the rest.

- ▸ Focus on what you are doing. Your opponents are more afraid of you than you are of them.

You will perform your best when you are relaxed, focused, mindful, and believe in yourself. When you are closest to your goal, be cautious and know that it may be your toughest moment. Here is how to develop a killer instinct:

DEVELOP YOUR KILLER INSTINCT

- ► Do not get too comfortable when you are doing well. Stay aggressive. Fight moment to moment.
- ► When you are doing very well, continue to challenge yourself so as not to become complacent.
- ► If your activation level drops, increase it and get pumped.

Unlike fear, physical pain is something you cannot ignore, but psychological pain is deceptive. Fear is insidious. It seeps into your mind when you least expect it. Yet, fear cannot take you down if you do not let it. Negativity requires an inflexible mindset and a lack of focus. If you remain mindful, you wear a suit of armor that cannot be pierced.

Although your fear may seem insurmountable at the time, keeping mindful of the present will allow you to look beyond your anxiety. If you focus on the moment your path will not seem so dreary. For example, if you are anxious about competing in a martial arts tournament, take a few seconds to use your visualization skills to imagine how you will feel when you have successfully done your best. Even though this is future-oriented, you are mindfully preparing yourself for the outcome of your competition. No one but you can cause debilitating anxiety.

Each week write down two of your fears so they cannot catch you by surprise. For me, that would include fear of heights and fear of failure. Simply by acknowledging these fears, I cannot be caught off guard by them. I know not to traverse a rope bridge without a lot of mental preparation. I also understand that if fear of failure stands in my way, then it is time for a change. Rather than fearing failure, I weigh the consequences of an assertive act, and if the gamble is warranted, I take a shot. If not, I adjust. By being proactive, even if I fail, I know that I tried.

The most difficult part of mindfulness is remembering to use it. It is easy to lose yourself in your fears. Although fear is debilitating, chronic worry, stress, and negativity are also emotional saboteurs. The same mindfulness that you use to combat fear will defeat these as well. Recognize signs and symptoms of over-activation and under-arousal caused by these emotions, then make the appropriate adjustments. Once again, mindfulness allows you to make systematic responses.

Try this:

STRATEGIES FOR REMEMBERING MINDFULNESS

1. Make a list of the things that make you scared or nervous.

2. Think about a time when everything was right in your life such as a moment of perfect peace or exhilaration.

3. Conjure up those thoughts and feelings of perfection.

4. During moments of fear or anxiety, bring back those thoughts and feelings of perfection into your life.

Anger

Usually anger is a negative emotional response to a stressful situation. Anger causes increased arousal, aggression, frustration, displeasure, and a need to retaliate. While its intensity varies, anger continuums can range from irritated to rage to fury. Whereas irritation and annoyance represent forms of mild anger, strongly emotional and energetic anger is known as rage. Expressed anger is exhibited in temper tantrums, cursing, and screaming, while suppressed anger consumes you with negative thoughts and images. Uncontrolled anger hurts your performance because it raises your activation beyond optimal levels. Remain mindful and you control your anger.

To control your anger:

STRATEGIES FOR CONTROLLING YOUR ANGER

► Change your anger into a laser-like focus.

► Change accompanying negative thoughts to positive ones.

► Break the anger pattern immediately. Do not let it get the best of you. Use a relaxation strategy to regain control.

▸ Think back to a time when anger hurt your performance. Use this image to strategize how you will quell your anger response the next time.

———————————————

Mood

Your mood is a transient, temporary emotional state or attitude. It fluctuates depending on your circumstances. Your mood depends on internal factors and external experiences. Your mood depends on tension-anxiety, depression-dejection, anger-hostility, vigor-activity, fatigue-inertia, and confusion-bewilderment. Recall the last time you were in a great mood. Recreate those thoughts and feelings so that you can return there. If you remain mindful, you are in control of your mood.

Creativity

Creativity is fun. Mindful people are creative because they are always observant. If you can be flexible you can be creative. Learn to adjust. Flexible people change strategies according to what works for them. If you come up with something only you can do, do it. Do not be afraid to challenge the status quo. Be yourself and do what works for you.

Preparing for Your Mind/Body Experience

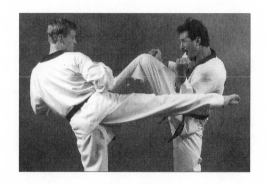

CHAPTER 4

Preparing for Your
✴ Mind/Body Experience ✴

Focused Effort

Without a strong body, your mind has no vehicle in which to express itself. Without a strong mind, your body cannot behave in a healthy manner. Balance is the key here. You must train your mind and body together. The motivation that you will need comes from within. Your purpose and inspiration combine with enthusiasm to help you reach your goals. When you are mindful, your enthusiasm is in line with your goals and ideals, and this combination makes for training and martial arts performance that is powerful regardless of your mood or what kind of day you are having.

Your motivation, however, must be yours alone. Copying someone else's martial arts training or performance will not work. A burning desire cannot be manufactured; it must be real and come from inside you and you alone. Your goals must fit into your scheme of thinking, behaving, and acting. If the goals are not yours, in time they will disappear. For some, this motivation seems to come quite naturally. For most it requires a lot of work, trial, tribulation, pain, and persistence.

With that said, stretch your comfort zone. Struggle to get ahead and be willing to pay a price. But be mindful just the same. If you listen closely to rock-and-roll, you will notice that the notes are all the same. Maybe a few changes from song to song, such as a few bars, a few breaks, and a few bridges thrown in here or there. So what is the difference? Feeling! When you pursue a dream, you are motivated and you feel it—so will others. Challenges, heartbreak, and securing a few victories along the way can keep you motivated to pursue your dream.

Re-evaluating Goals

Mindfulness as I see it does not mean sitting in meditation eight hours a day. You need to experience variety. Open yourself to multitudes of experiences that will provide you with a strong foundation. The more you experience the more you will understand, and nothing will rock you.

During my RAAM training, slowly but surely, my six hours of daily physical training began to take its toll on my body. My first painful experience was plantar fasciitis and a heel spur, which translated into debilitating heel pain. As if that was not enough, hip tendinitis reared its ugly head from thousands of pedal strokes a day. At first I ignored the pain and continued training. Soon, the symptoms worsened and I consulted M.D.'s, physical therapists, and chiropractors. The M.D.'s gave me anti-inflammatory injections and physical therapists and chiropractors taught me stretching exercises, but nothing worked. The pain subsided only when I cut back on my activity. So I dropped my exercise from six to three hours a day and rearranged my priorities. Rather than spend three hours on my bike and climbing a stair machine, I spent 45 minutes on my bike, 45 minutes on my stair climber, and 45 minutes teaching my kids tennis. Although my injuries did not heal, the pain lessened. Training six hours a day was a relic from my athletic years when it was a badge of honor to workout like an animal. With my new training protocol, my goal was to spend the least amount of time training, and yet gain maximum results—a far cry from the days when I would not pedal into my driveway until I had been on the road for six hours. My goals needed to be re-evaluated so I took control. If you are in a place with your training that you do not want to be or cannot be, take the time to re-evaluate your goals and try to experience new things.

Breathe

Hippocrates said that a patient should be at the helm of his or her own healing. Herbert Benson, a Harvard cardiologist, went on to say, "Ideally medicine should be a three-legged stool, with the legs of surgery and pharmaceuticals balanced with spiritual self-care, such as meditation or prayer. Yet often this third leg is missing."

Benson asserts that sixty to ninety percent of all illness is brought on by stress. According to Dr. Benson, "Reciting a prayer, focusing on a particular image, word, or physical motion (like the heel-to-toe rocking that Orthodox Jews do during worship) is a balm for an amazing number of ailments."

Stress-related disorders have long been eased by spiritual practice. During prayer, breathing is long and deep, the heartbeats are slower and the mind is focused.

It has been found that breathing is a natural stress-buster. You do it all the time, so why not use it to your advantage. You may not notice that you inhale and exhale at least fifteen thousand times each day. Yet if you run after a bus or swim the length of a pool under water, suddenly you realize how breathing, or the lack thereof, can affect every cell in your body. Shallow, rapid breathing can trigger the fight-or-flight response. However, if you take long deep breaths and focus on your breathing, you will relax.

A variety of gurus teach different breathing skills and drills. One strategy for example, teaches you to breathe in through one nostril and out the other. While another instructs you to focus on the temperature and vibration of the air as it passes through your nasal passages. Whatever way you choose to do it, breathing is a first step in your mind/body connection.

STRESS CONTROL BREATHING

When you are anxious, your body prepares for a crisis. Blood is quickly transported to your muscles for fight-or-flight. Your blood pressure and heart rate increase, and, in order to get the oxygen you need, you unconsciously breathe faster. As you exhale you quickly release carbon dioxide which changes your blood pH. This keeps your blood from efficiently getting oxygen to your brain, muscles, and organs.

When you inhale and exhale impulsively, you hyperventilate. If you are anxious all day long, you may be in a constant state of hyperventilation. You may even be hyperventilating at this very moment. The lower lobes of your lungs lie below your chest. Breathe deeply and allow air to fill this area. This is diaphragmatic breathing. It is much different from the shallow breathing caused by anxiety, and it will relax you.

Muscle tension, especially tight abdominal muscles, constrict your diaphragm and restricts your breathing. Take a deep breath from your belly. This short circuits your sympathetic nervous system and lessens your stress reaction. Your heart rate and blood pressure will automatically drop. Focus on your breathing. Just by altering your attention, you can decrease your anxiety.

Your lower lungs inflate with less effort than your upper lungs. Most people do not know how to take advantage of this. Count your inhalations. You probably inhale about twenty times per minute. Now, try to fill your lungs by taking in more air with each breath. This will cause you to breathe slower. Breathing slowly and smoothly helps stabilize your blood pH allowing oxygen to more readily reach your brain and organs. Belly breathers average eight to fourteen inhalations per minute.

HOW TO BREATHE

There are a few different ways to breathe. Most folks breathe so that when they inhale their chest expands while their abdomen contracts. This is termed thoracic breathing. Another way of breathing is reverse breathing. When you breathe this way your abdomen expands when you inhale and contracts when you exhale. Neither of these patterns is as healthy as diaphragmatic breathing which allows the air in the bottom of your lungs to be efficiently transported out and replaced by fresh air.

Breathing is subtle, yet quite extraordinary. Although breathing is normally involuntary, an act of will can slow it down or speed it up. Breathing is a present-time, mindful process. You cannot be enjoying fond memories or planning your future when you are contemplating your breath. Observe your breath, and you are automatically in the present.

As you focus on your breath, you can try different breathing strategies. One breathing strategy is to mindfully pay attention to the sensations as air passes through your nostrils. Inhale through your nose. Notice the point just inside your nose where you have the most powerful sensation of airflow. Then exhale and feel the sensation again. Focus your attention on this spot. Similar to a martial artist gazing at the solar plexus of the opponent and seeing the adversary's entire body with peripheral vision, you should focus on this spot and watch the rest of your breath go in and out. Just breathe naturally and mindfully watch your breath. You will notice sometimes it slows, speeds up, or is deep, short, or choppy. Just observe and be mindful of how thoughts inadvertently affect your breathing. Each time, though, be sure to come back to the object of your focus—your breath.

Another strategy that you can try is the following. At the beginning of your inhalation, follow your breath with your mind just for that inhalation. Then, at the start of your exhalation, follow your breath just for that exhalation. Focus on a single breath cycle. Be mindful of your breathing at that moment. Forget about the last breath, and do not think about the next one. Just exist in the moment.

Heart Rate Response and Mind/Body Training

The pace of your heart is unique to your body. It is self-regulating. You do not have to do a thing, yet it keeps beating and maintains its own rhythm to keep you alive. Yet, there are a variety of psychological and physiological factors that affect your heart rate.

Your hormonal responses, central nervous system (CNS), and autonomic nervous system (ANS) can affect the speed and rhythm of your heart. Your hormones send chemicals into your blood that affect your heart's pace. Your heart also beats faster or slower depending on how your nerves stimulate it.

While reading this passage, mindfully imagine your spouse or a good friend tapping you on your shoulder or think back to when you stepped into the ring for the first time. Your heart raced uncontrollably. External stimulus from your nerves or hormones can automatically speed up your heart rate. Mindfulness allows you to predict and override a conditioned physiological response. Through mindful practice you can regulate your heart rate when you are threatened. You can mindfully slow it down so that you will be able relax and handle any situation appropriately.

Such mindfulness is enhanced if you understand the physiology of your brain to heart connection. The medulla of your brain is your control center for your heart rate. It either speeds or slows your beats per minute. Your ANS has two components: Your sympathetic nervous system (SNS) and parasympathetic nervous system (PNS). Your SNS speeds your heart rate by releasing hormones and chemicals called norepinephrine, epinephrine, and catecholamines. When your heart races uncontrollably you experience tachycardia. There is no cardiovascular benefit to your body when your SNS increases your heart rate. It is simply your hormones sending stimulating chemicals to your heart, and nerves directly affecting your heart to respond to an emergency situation.

Your PNS is in your brain stem. This is the area that slows your heart rate. A chemical that your PNS releases to slow your heart rate is called acetylcholine. When your heart rate slows, you experience bradycardia. Mind/body technicians are famous for slowing their heart rates. Some yogis can slow their heart rates to the less than twenty beats per minute. The famous magician, Harry Houdini was able to survive in a coffin-sized airtight box for hours in this state.

Your nerves and hormones together regulate your heart rate when you are moving and when you are still. As you begin training, your heart rate speeds up because your PNS is inhibited. That is, the mechanisms that slow your heart are essentially turned off, and your beats per minute (bpm) naturally increases.

Some of the other factors that can affect the pace of your heart include blood sugar levels, different foods, lack of sleep, anxiety, fear, and anger. Feelings of peace, love, and compassion lower heart rates while nervousness, aggression, and trepidation speed it up. Chronic nervousness, sometimes referred to as trait anxiety, can cause your heart rate to remain elevated for extended periods of time. This is where mindfulness comes in. Meditation and relaxation techniques have proven successful in reducing chronic tachycardia caused by such things as trait anxiety.

Most people believe that the better shape you are in, the slower your heart rate, right? Not necessarily. Professional tennis player Bjorn Borg owned a resting heart rate of 35 bpm's. Now that makes sense because Borg was an elite athlete. However, Olympic marathon superstar, Frank Shorter's resting heart rate was 75 bpm's. Your genes account for about 50 percent of what your maximum heart rate will turn out to be. Smaller hearts beat faster than larger ones. In general, the more fit you are, the stronger your heartbeat, the more blood you pump with each beat. Meaning, the better shape you are in, the longer and stronger your heart will beat.

Environmental factors can also affect your heart rate. For example if you are tired, on medication, under stress, at high altitude, or in high humidity, your heart rate may change. Therefore, be mindful of environmental factors.

During your martial arts training, your CNS is the most influential factor determining your heart rate. When you tie your dobok, your CNS sends messages to your medulla to prepare for activity. Suddenly, your heart rate increases even before you step onto the mat. Just by anticipating a workout, your heart rate can increase as much as 100 percent. Mindfulness provides you with the tools to decrease your heart rate and improve your martial arts performance.

Physiology and Mind/Body

Mindfulness affects your thoughts and your thoughts control your body. Your thoughts and feelings influence your body through your nervous and circulatory system. This is how your brain communicates with your body. Your nervous system acts as a conduit between your brain and body by sending nervous impulses into your muscles and tissues. Your entire body is wired to your brain. These messages extend into your immune system, bone marrow, thymus, spleen, lymph nodes, endocrine system, bones, muscles, internal organs, and the walls of your veins and arteries.

Your brain also manufactures thousands of different chemicals and releases them into your bloodstream. The cells of your body receive these chemicals and respond accordingly. Theoretically, you can mindfully control these chemicals thus influencing the activity and behavior of your tissues.

Mindfulness provides you with more power over your body than you can imagine. By mindfully quieting your stress-response or sending blood to your hands and feet by taking control of your sympathetic nervous system, you will naturally calm your emotions. Through practice of mindfulness you can gain a greater awareness of your physiology, which, in turn, allows you to control your body.

PLACEBO EFFECT

Your mind can have an incredible placebo effect on your body. In 1957 the *Journal of Projective Techniques* reported an example of the placebo power of your mind/body. The subject was a man with metastatic cancer and tumors that had spread throughout his body. He tried every available form of medicine, yet his condition had hopelessly deteriorated. He was bedridden and his doctors agreed he could only live a few days longer. It was at this time of his illness that the man heard about a new experimental drug to cure cancer and he asked to be used as a guinea pig during the experimental trials. Although his doctors felt it was a lost cause, they gave him the drug. The tumors shrunk dramatically and the patient was released from the hospital. Two months later, the patient heard that the drug was proven ineffective. Within days his fatal tumors returned. His doctors, realizing the power of the placebo, provided the patient with a more potent form of the drug (they injected him with water). His tumors once again shrank dramatically. He remained stable for several months until he saw a news report on television that said his drug was useless. He died two days later.

Mindfulness allows for a strong connection between your mind body. Mindful observation and visualization can be successfully used to help you overcome many obstacles.

THE STRESS RESPONSE

If you are threatened by a real or imagined danger, your body responds. The intensity or subtlety of the response depends on the magnitude of the perceived threat. This fight-or-flight reaction, the stress response, has the beneficial effect of preparing your body to function at a higher level of efficiency for a short duration of time during a self-defense situation or martial arts performance. Such physiological responses include:

- Increased blood pressure
- Increased respiratory rate
- Increased heart rate
- Increased oxygen consumption (burning of fuel)
- Increased blood flow to skeletal muscles
- Increased perspiration
- Increased muscle tone

Regular stimulation of these stress responses can decrease immune function and lead to chronic stress related problems.

THE RELAXATION RESPONSE

Harvard cardiologist Herbert Benson studied the effects of a meditation technique called the relaxation response. This relaxed and yet focused altered state of consciousness proved to be beneficial in a variety of ways. Specifically, the benefits of the relaxation response countered or balanced the negative effects of the stress response. Relaxation responses include:

- Reduced blood pressure
- Reduced respiratory rate
- Reduced heart rate
- Reduced oxygen consumption (burning of fuel)
- Reduced blood flow to skeletal muscles

‣ Reduced perspiration

‣ Reduced muscle tension

The relaxation response is not a technique. It is a state that the body enters during mindful practice. There are strategies other than meditation that you can use to elicit the beneficial effects of the relaxation response. Such techniques are listed below.

STRATEGIES FOR RELAXATION RESPONSES

‣ **Autogenic Training.** Autogenic training is a combination of self-suggestion and imagery. Practice of autogenic training includes repeating phrases to yourself such as "I am relaxed and calm, and my body tingles." You then focus on a particular body part and send calming energy into that area to relax it.

‣ **Breathing.** Breathing techniques can be used in combination with autogenic training and meditation or by themselves. Deep breathing contributes to healing and increased energy. Use of deep diaphragmatic breathing will relax your body and release pain. Breathing can also be used to increase speed and power by focusing your exhalation through pursed lips.

‣ **Hypnosis.** Hypnosis is not magic, it is simply a condition of heightened concentration. As in many other strategies, hypnosis requires relaxation and concentration to bring about an extraordinary focus. Some people use hypnosis to influence their mind/body.

‣ **Biofeedback.** Biofeedback uses special instrumentation to tell you what is going on in your body. These instruments amplify signals that you may not otherwise notice. EMG biofeedback measures electrical activity in your muscles. During a biofeedback session a sensor may be placed on your forehead; as you relax, a loud beep will get softer and softer until you are completely relaxed and the beep stops.

You can use less sophisticated techniques to measure you body's relaxation state, such as a thermometer. A thermometer measures heat, so the greater the temperature, the more blood flow there is in your body, and the more relaxed you are. Other simpler biofeedback mechanisms include being mindful of your heart rate and respiration to measure your anxiety or activation.

Once you can see that if you are mindful to what is happening inside your body, you have the ability to change it. When we were children we learned how to walk and talk by instinctively using feedback mechanisms. Such mechanisms are simply an internal manifestation of the feedback process.

Biofeedback works best when you intend to regulate some variable, but then remain relaxed about whether or not it changes. It is this same attitude that you should use when you practice mindfulness and martial arts. You exist in the moment visualizing your results, but you do not obsess about the outcome.

Mind/Body Competition

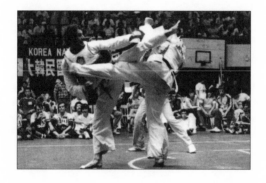

CHAPTER 5

✳ Mind/Body Competition ✳

Sports Performance

Would it not be great if you could recapture and bottle the wonderful feelings and thoughts you had immediately after you completed your first martial arts training session? How about recapturing confident feelings and thoughts you had when you were naturally relaxed and focused, knowing you would win your first martial arts tournament? Would not it be great if you could experience these thoughts and feelings consistently? Do you think such resourceful feelings and thoughts would improve your martial arts performance? Count on it!

SPORTS COMPETITION AND MINDFULNESS

In America we tend to exhibit a win-at-all-costs ideal. This American ideal does not work in your best interest. Taoist thought states, "Do not seek victory in contention, for where there is no contention, there is neither victory nor defeat, the supple willow does not contend against the storm yet it survives." This premise provides an insight that is more balanced and healthy. By looking at a martial arts competition or situation from this perspective, you can see that instead of fighting so that you do not lose, you can free yourself to let yourself win.

Some people like to train for the sake of training; others enjoy training for contests. Spending hours honing movements, bending knees, and following through can be either meaningful or painfully boring—depending on your perspective. Potential martial arts athletes who disdain practice may achieve a modicum of success, but mindful practice is what makes champions.

Olympic Taekwondo champions spend hours whittling their bodies into condition. Their commitment to training is strengthened by daily short-term achievements. They understand that stronger, more agile athletes that have more endurance are superior competitors. To these Olympic champions, a disciplined, mindful practice schedule is a normal part of their every day routine. The daily ritual of repetitive practice is mindful training. It sharpens your mind/body. The process of such training is just as important as the product.

There are other ways to practice than spending monotonous hours in a gym. A friend and sparring partner, Raymond McCallum, a Professional Karate Association full contact champion, was rarely seen in a gym. While the rest of us were busy skipping rope and lifting weights, Ray was riding his Harley. Yet every time Ray stepped into the ring, he was focused. He was relaxed and in the zone. Competition itself was his mindful training.

Music is another way to bring mindfulness and excitement into an otherwise lackluster training session. Music inspires. Your favorite tunes can psyche you to a frenzy and increase your activation. Listening to your preferred CD or audio tape while visualizing a perfect practice session can set the tone for what may have been an otherwise monotonous workout. The nice thing about music is that you can listen in the car, during idle moments at home, or on your way to a tournament. Then during your martial arts workout or performance you can recreate the beat in your mind.

When you started your martial arts training, you did not realize the profound knowledge that exercise and competition provide. Learning martial arts requires mindfulness and mindfulness carries over into every aspect of your life. This, in turn, leads to increased mind/body development.

The Science Behind Mindfulness in Sports

Your attitudes and cognition have biological consequences. Even small and seemingly innocuous attitudes affect your stress hormones, which then alter your immune and endocrine systems. Long-term, chronic stress increases your heart rate, blood pressure, muscle tension, and blood sugar levels. Sometimes this red-alert status does not go away, and your organ systems remain in a heightened state. Such conditions of prolonged stress can bring about side effects like irritable bowel syndrome and migraine headaches to name a few.

SPORT MINDFULNESS

As a martial artist, you have been in the heat of battle. If your body and your mind are going in different directions, it is tough to reach your mind/body goals. By transferring the mindfulness you practice during your martial arts to your daily routine you can experience the mind/body connection all the time.

When you compete against yourself, there is no ego. Do not be so invested in your own success. Success will happen if you remain mindful and let it. Competition breeds pressure. Competitive pressures bring butterflies and muscle tension. Do not worry, however, because these are natural responses, especially if the event at hand means a lot to you. Even if you are mindful, you cannot help but feel exhilarated by competition, so allow it to enhance your martial arts performance rather than inhibit it. Improve your focus and raise the bar to higher standards. While others are overwhelmed by stress, anxiety, and fear your martial arts performance will remain uninhibited. Be careful, though. The increase in activation caused by fear, anxiety, and worry can over-arouse you and hurt your performance. These negative emotions steal energy if you let them. That is why mindfulness is a key ingredient. Look at competitive pressure objectively. Channel increased activation into your performance outcome, and guard against negative emotional arousal.

Harness your activation energy, and quell negative emotions. Believe in yourself when you step in the ring and know inside that nervous energy is a natural part of your performance. Trust your preparation. Win your internal war by remaining focused and welcoming uncertainty with excitement. When you press too hard, your physiology will overload, and your heart rate and blood pressure will skyrocket. Instead, be mindful.

Develop a well thought-out preparation strategy. That way, you can remain mindful and make rapid and accurate decisions under fire and adjust to unexpected situations easily.

Competition should neither threaten your self-esteem nor make you angry. Although competition is not an end, it is fun and challenging. Competition has ups and downs, positives and negatives. Competing exposes your weaknesses and develops your strengths, while helping you stretch your limits. It makes you stronger and teaches you to focus and to solve problems. It enhances your confidence and self-esteem. Just be sure not to get too serious. Keep it fun, never give up, believe in yourself, and always remain mindful.

SELF-AWARENESS IS MINDFULNESS

Whether you hope to win a martial arts tournament or be your best you need self-awareness. Even though you may ponder ways to win, more importantly, you must know yourself so you can improve. Remaining mindful before your event profoundly affects your subsequent performance. You are conditioned. Maximize yourself.

Your mindfulness affects how you think and feel, just as your thoughts and feelings moderate your behavior. You may do well when you are highly activated or very relaxed. Notice and record the relationship between your activation level and your performance:

- Rate how you performed on a scale of 1–10.
- Estimate your activation level, confidence, and focus on scales from 1–10.
- Include ratings both before and after competition.

After awhile, you will notice that patterns become visible. Mindfulness of your thoughts, feelings, and actions help you replicate desirable performances. Self-awareness is mindfulness.

Concentration and Mindfulness in Martial Arts Activity

In previous chapters, I have spoken of the difference between concentration and mindfulness. In competition each has its role and their relationship is intricate and important. Concentration is often called focus. It requires your mind to remain on a static point. Concentration is laser-like and can be developed by sheer, unrelenting willpower.

Mindfulness is different. It is sensitive. It notices things. During your martial arts, mindfulness and concentration are partners. Mindfulness provides you with the power to keep your attention pinned to the cues necessary to achieve peak performance. Mindfulness picks the object of your attention and notices when your focus has gone astray. Concentration is the workhorse while mindfulness keeps you steady. If either of these is weak, your sports performance deteriorates.

Concentration focuses single-mindedly on one cue without interruption. Concentration is your tool to focus. When you are focused, you do not think about dinner or how much you want to win. Mindfulness tells you how to use that tool. Mindfulness is there to notice. It is not required to focus; instead, it sees everything peripherally and objectively. Mindfulness notices everything, and it does not categorize. Distractions are seen with the same attention as performance cues. When you are mindful, your attention flows and shifts and finally focuses on the object of your concentration.

Unlike concentration, mindfulness does not improve by force or willpower. Mindfulness is improved by relaxation, settling down, and letting go. Mindfulness sees your performance objectively, exactly as it is, not what you hoped it would be, it sees whatever is there. Mindfulness is not trying, because there is no goal. When you are mindful you are looking at everything as if for the first time—innocent, with a sense of wonder. Mindfulness looks at each moment as if it were the only moment.

While concentration is exclusive, mindfulness is all-encompassing. Concentration focuses on one item and ignores everything else. Mindfulness stands back from the focus of attention and watches with a broad brush, quick to notice any change that occurs. For example, if you find yourself in a street defense situation and you are attacked, you will see only your assailant. That is, until his partner grabs you from behind. Mindfulness stands back, aware of the attacker in the front, and behind. Mindfulness notices your mental distraction and redirects your attention back to defending against the most immediate danger.

Mindfulness is more difficult to cultivate than concentration because it is similar to an overseer. Concentration is merely focusing on the cue at hand. It does not, however, direct what it sees. Mindfulness is constantly responsible for assimilating and directing your attention appropriately.

Patience and awareness are the keys to improved mindfulness as well as simple acceptance. Concentration and mindfulness go hand-in-hand for improved performance. Ideally, mindfulness directs your concentration. Mindfulness is the boss, and concentration does the work. Mindfulness provides you with the foundation for deeper concentration.

If you are mindful, your concentration will develop naturally. The more you develop your ability to notice, the more quickly you perceive distractions and return to your focus. As your concentration improves so, too, does your mindfulness. The more focused you are, the less chance there is of becoming distracted. You will note the distraction and return to your focus. Mindfulness and concentration balance and support each other.

Competition Anxiety

If, during a martial arts competition, your mind becomes wild and agitated, breathe a few quick breaths to re-establish mindfulness. Close your mouth and pull air in strongly through your nose and exhale the same way. This increases the air flow sensation inside your nostrils and gives you something on which to focus.

When it is important for you to maintain your focus, count your breaths. Your breathing cadence slows and becomes lighter. Say "in" when you inhale, and "ahh" when you exhale. Soon your breath becomes light and gentle, so much so that there seems little difference between your inhalation and exhalation. They blend. Notice your natural sensation of breathing. Inhalation transitions to exhalation. One breath follows the next in an eternal cycle. This is your signal that your focus is pure.

During your bout, negative thoughts may hang on. Make it a ritual to dismiss negative thoughts when your match begins. At first your thought process will not obey, but after awhile, your mind learns not to obsess while you are on the competition floor. This is a perfect case of classical conditioning; your mindfulness remains on the lookout for negativity and squashes it.

Conversely, anger, fear, and anxiety can break your concentration if your mindfulness is weak. When fear wells up, your concentration locks onto it and fear pulls energy away from your task. Allow your mindfulness to notice this attention glitch and return you to the proper focus. Your mindfulness sweeps this unwanted emotion under the rug. When negativity again rears its ugly head, mindfulness is there to save the day.

Mindful martial artists have a great sense of humor; they have learned to laugh at their failures. Elite martial artists remain relaxed during their performances. You need to do the same. Do not be too serious. Do not try too hard. Laugh a little. Loosen up and learn to go with whatever happens.

ROLE MODELS

The Eastern approach to training requires living in the present. Exercise is not just a habit. Working out is an exercise in mindfulness. Workouts meant much more than bigger arms or passing time. Ancient martial artists endured hours of intense physical pain as an end in itself. They practiced sharpening their minds. Training changed their lives. Perfecting a movement was a doorway to the zone. At completion, there was a sense of accomplishment and well-being.

When I was a youngster, a friend and I sneaked over the barbed-wire fence of our army base in Okinawa and walked several miles to a karate school located in the ground floor of a hotel in an impoverished Okinawan village. Two weeks after we joined, my buddy quit so I made the pilgrimage alone each night. I was captivated by the discipline. Few Americans trained in our Okinawan dojo (karate school). Not because of price (it cost an exorbitant six dollars per month) or because there was a language barrier. For many Americans, performing the same program night after night, year after year, was tedious. My Okinawan classmates did not seem to mind. They reveled in discipline. For them karate was an art.

At exactly seven o'clock in the evening our sensei (instructor) would line us up. We then dropped to our knees and bowed saying in unison, *Onee guy etashi mas,* ("Please show me the way"). This fifteen-second ceremony cleared our minds and prepared us for training. Each workout required us to concentrate fully. At exactly nine o'clock we bowed saying, *Arrigato gozai mashta* ("Thank you for showing me the way"). This moment symbolized a return to world outside of the training hall.

A year into my training, the dojo was closed several consecutive nights without explanation. The sensei's son, Zenpo Shimabuku, opened the sliding glass doors to explain to us that his 80-year-old father had died while demonstrating kicking techniques in Japan. The Master's appendix ruptured, but he did not take the time to seek medical attention.

The Shimabuku's and my Okinawan classmates were fun-loving, yet centered people. They possessed an inner stillness. Even when Mother Nature unleashed devastating typhoons that demolished their homes they began rebuilding the next day. The Okinawans exemplified mindfulness. Discomfort was a prerequisite for survival. They seemed mindful of their activity and they were always smiling.

Mind/Body and Speed/Power

Martial arts require speed, flexibility, endurance, strength, and power. The faster, stronger, and more flexible you are and the more stamina you possess, the better your chances are of winning. Although you may develop these attributes through training and competition, it is also essential to develop a relaxed and focused mindset. There are a few competitors who have never thought about the benefits of mindfulness. Maybe you are one of them.

Some martial artists do not hoist weights or jog. They never lift a finger out of the dojo to improve their in-the-ring performance. Rather, their power comes from within—a relaxed mindset. Since power is a function of speed and strength, they remain focused on speed. They developed a whip-like move to create power in their technique. These athletes, however, will never realize their full power. Strength is the other half of the power equation. It is a combination of both speed and strength that provide ultimate power.

Strength without relaxation produces mechanical, lackluster movement. On the other hand, relaxation without strength manifests as aesthetically pleasing, but powerless. You can achieve optimum martial arts performance by training your muscles and your mind simultaneously. An external martial artist who takes time to develop his or her mind/body can increase both speed and power. If a mind/body martial artist develops his or her physical attributes, he or she will exhibit greater power.

External martial artists train their muscles, tendons, and bones, while internal martial artists train their synapses, confidence, and mindset. Mindfulness is a luxury you carry with you for life. The sooner you develop it, the greater your rewards.

If your external martial arts goal is to enhance your power, then you should know that there is an inverse relationship between speed and force. In other words, if you are relaxed, you can move quickly. The more force you put behind your movement, the slower you will be. Therefore, you must develop both speed and force. If you increase your speed and force, your power will improve incrementally. It does not matter which comes first, speed or force. Multiply speed and force and you produce power.

Whether you develop your psyche or put all of your energy into maximizing your external strengths does not matter. Your ultimate goal is to maximize the product of both your physical technique and your mindfulness. Considering the benefits of mind/body puts you on the right track. Awareness of where you would like to be will propel you to your goal.

In essence, the mind/body martial artist is a better more complete athlete. He or she understands the value of relaxation and force to increase speed and power. Yet, mind/body martial artists understand that power is not everything. Power without psyche is a waste. Mindfulness focuses your energy like a laser. It is the combination of mind/body and force that will power your ultimate performance. Spend time developing mindfulness and watch your power grow.

You may wonder what happens to your speed, force, and power as you grow older. As you age, you lose fast-twitch muscle fibers and your reaction time slows. Your aerobic power decreases, and you may feel a twinge of arthritis. That is why it is so crucial to improve your mindfulness. Although your speed, force, and power may decline and cause you to lose a step or two, possessing mindfulness in your twilight years more than compensates.

MIND/BODY MARTIAL ARTS

Some traditional mind/body activities have lost their innocence and become competitive. That is, the mind/body connection has disappeared. Karate practiced as an art is a mind/body experience, but when martial artists step into the competitive arena, the mind/body disappears with the first punch. Especially in professional martial arts. When I fought my first professional full contact fight on ESPN, there was no such thing as honor and sportsmanship. What mattered was winning, at all costs.

In the Taekwondo ring however, there continues to be a mind/body approach to competition. Taekwondo coaches teach their charges that once they retire from competition, they may continue a mind/body legacy in their art. Therefore, pick and choose your mind/body sports with an eye toward the ultimate purpose for your training.

Martial Arts Breathing

Mindful breathing keeps you in touch with your body so you perform better. Breathing is one of your best biofeedback mechanisms. Most people worry about getting as much oxygen into their bodies as possible so they can finish their bout. If however you focus on your process of breathing, you can tune into your body and be mindful of your martial arts performance.

During high intensity martial arts activity, inhale through your nose and mouth to get as much oxygen as possible to your working muscles. Then exhale through your mouth only and contract your intercostal muscles around the lower part of your ribcage, along with your abdominal muscles to allow carbon dioxide to be drawn out of your body. This allows your diaphragm to lift, and decreases erratic breathing patterns. Staccato type breathing stimulates your sympathetic nervous system and increases your heart rate. A rapid heart rate wastes energy and inhibits your mind/body experience as well as your mindfulness.

To find the proper breathing rhythm for your art, exhale through pursed lips until you discover your natural inhalation-exhalation cycle. Controlling and extending your exhalation process helps to remove carbon dioxide more efficiently. After a controlled exhalation, passively inhale a deep, oxygen-filled breath to increase nutrients to your muscles. Your aerobic power will increase, and ultimately so will your overall martial arts performance.

Remember when your coaches told you to relax, but that was easier said than done? Proper breathing is your first step. Diaphragmatic breathing relaxes you when you feel the jitters. To gain better control of your breathing skills practice breathing drills throughout practice and during your performance. Controlled breathing moderates your heart rate and improves your circulation. A deep cleansing breath clears you mind. If at any time during your practice session you need to collect yourself, it is the perfect time for diaphragmatic breathing. At the culmination of your practice or performance, use breathing to cool you down and prepare you to re-enter the real world.

You know how important relaxation is for exemplary performance. Inflexible, clenched-fisted determination will not improve your performance. Mindfulness will. Before you kick a field goal, putt a golf ball, throw a pitch, swing a bat, field a ball, throw a punch, or shoot a free throw, relaxation is a must—and it all begins with breathing. Start your breath from a position three inches below your naval. Breathe in through your nose and let air fill your abdomen all the way into your chest. Take about five seconds to inhale until your lungs feel full and hold it for two seconds. Then, exhale slowly to an eight count. Relax all of your muscles and focus on your breath. Continue this until there is no unnecessary tension in your body.

STRATEGIES FOR MINDFUL BREATHING

▸ Get into the habit of doing your breathing exercises as a ritual during certain times of your practice and performance. When you practice breathing at home, do it at a regular time and place. Your body will look forward to this respite, and your mind will associate this with a time for absolute mindfulness.

▸ If you are practicing your breathing at home, find a quiet, comfortable place and loosen your clothing.

▸ If you lie down, be sure you do not fall asleep. Have an alarm clock prepared just in case.

▸ Clear your mind and begin to focus only on your breathing. Exist in the moment. Breathing is your only priority and your only interest.

Mentally Preparing for Competition

Getting psyched is extremely important to exemplary achievement. Knowing when to turn it on will help you be your best. Evander Holyfield does not hold back when he throws a punch. World Karate Champion, Bill Wallace pummels opponents with vicious left foot attacks. Both of these champions summon all of their physical and mental strength to win, yet their emotions hardly enter the ring. Punching and kicking is their craft, and they are workmanlike in their devastation.

Preparing for a martial arts tournament requires a tremendous amount of mindfulness. During idle moments your attention can shift to your upcoming contest. Your stomach rumbles, muscles tighten, and palms sweat. This fight-or-flight response can be is distressing. Would-be competitors can have difficulty handling tension. Their bodies become ill, and they can injure themselves. They are simply not mindful of their emotions.

Such competitors may have been physically ready but not mentally fit. It is easy to exaggerate the caliber of adversaries or the magnitude of an event. Rather than viewing competition as win-lose or succeed-fail, approach each match with mindfulness. If you are mindful you can learn more about yourself in a single tournament than in six months of training. Competition brings out your best as well as your worst. Stay relaxed and mindful. Pay attention to how you move and how you react. Be mindful of everything and success will follow.

During a competitive martial arts tournament, spectators increase your activation by amplifying the urgency of your event. The better prepared you are, the more an audience will spur you on. Competition is electrifying. It puts you on the edge and allows you to transcend your limits. Give yourself an opportunity to be your best by allowing your mindfulness to focus your attention.

Emotions are a double-edged sword because they increase your intensity and multiply your chances for error. Counterproductive feelings, such as defensiveness and negative emotions, sabotage your performance and weaken you. During intense martial arts competition you may feel frustration and experience antagonism. That is why mindfulness is your key to emotional control. If you anticipate a difficult situation, plan a response and set limits on your emotional behavior. No matter how bad things become, acknowledge your opponent for issuing a challenge and promise yourself not to succumb. The tougher your opponent is, the more you will mature. If you can remain mindful under these conditions, you can handle anything.

You must also remember that you have no control over your opponent's personality or techniques, so focus on your performance. Develop a system. If your rival displays malevolence, ignore him or her. When your opponent rages, use his or her misplaced energy to fuel your tenacity and courage. Mindfulness forces negative emotions to take a back seat. It is impossible to be enraged and mindful at the same time.

In a martial arts tournament you may compete for only a short period of time in comparison to the total event. The remainder of your time is spent waiting. Use this time to prepare for your subsequent bout. Immediately begin to think about your next opponent. Do not exalt yourself until the tournament is finished. During the World Taekwondo Championships in Germany, I fought the defending heavyweight, Dirk Jung. He beat me in the finals of the Asian Games in Taiwan just two months earlier. He was primed to win a second straight World Championship in front of his home crowd in Stuttgart. The round before we fought, he had a ferocious fray with the Korean representative. Jung celebrated his conquest with a victory lap. He rejoiced and probably felt the battle was over. His body was in a recovery mode, leaving him too relaxed. It was difficult for him to regroup and be his emotional best for our fight. He lost his mindfulness. He lost the bout.

Do not permit a negative attitude to limit your performance. Hostility affects your confidence and concentration. Transform fear or anger into focused energy. Begin with relaxation and then follow with concentration. Mindfulness does not come fast or easy, mental preparation is a skill. If you try too hard, you will undermine your efforts. Ask yourself, "Why am I competing?"

Identify your mental toughness goals so that you know what it is that you are specifically attempting to achieve. Establish both martial arts performance objectives and outcome goals, then set short and long-term targets. Setting goals to improve your attitude provides direction and guides you on your journey. A proper attitude directs your attention toward accomplishing a task. Accomplishment that increases your self-esteem is not just about doing something, it is about the mindfulness to persist through pain, failure, and self-doubt.

Mindfulness improves your competitive martial arts performance. Whether you are a high-strung accountant or laid-back landscaper, when it comes to competition, everyone is the same. Everyone experiences pain as well as satisfaction. Competition is a privilege no matter where you have been, no matter who you are.

As you approach the final days before your martial arts event, nothing you do physically can help, but you can hurt your performance if you overtrain. Become mindful of your impending performance and sensitive to your body's signals. Focus on the task at hand. Tune into yourself with an energy that opens you to the possibility of your potential.

Barriers are mostly self-imposed. Maybe you are afraid of the physical discomfort required to win your event or maybe you know the bar will be raised for your next competition if you win this one. As your suppositions about your limits change, the limits themselves become altered. Your beliefs about yourself and your potential can change your reality.

I have seen martial artists of similar abilities perform at opposite ends of the spectrum. Although they had the same strength, endurance, and flexibility, one won and one lost. Mindfulness was the determining factor. Although motivation and drive may seem inborn, I do not believe they are. I believe that you can consciously develop psychological skills to enhance your martial arts performance:

- ▶ SELF-MOTIVATION. Your efforts must come from inside. If you are doing it for your sensei, partner, or your parents, that is not enough and it will not work.
- ▶ OVERCOME OBSTACLES. Remain calm and focused under fire. Allow pressure to fuel your performance. When adversity strikes, view it as a challenge to come back and overcome it.
- ▶ COMMIT YOURSELF. Make your training and performance a priority. Cut out unessential time wasters like watching too much television and mindless phone conversations, etc.
- ▶ POSITIVE FOCUS. Your choice is to complain about things you cannot change or be mindful of your progress. Remain positive and spend energy attending to those items within your control.

- ▸ DRIVE. Your desire to improve is based on your motivation to achieve. This all begins with a goal. Turn this goal into a burning desire. Think about your goal, mission, and purpose daily. Take tiny steps each day to reach your goal.
- ▸ REJUVENATE. Rise to the occasion no matter the circumstances. Energize yourself for peak performance. Generate optimal arousal via mindfulness.

As a competitor and advisor to athletes for over thirty years, I have seen the same problems over and over again: motivational problems, lack of confidence, anxiety, pre-performance nerves, fear of losing, and injury. Everyone wants to know the secret to mindfulness. When you observe high level martial arts athletes you understand there is no secret. It is a combination of relaxation and focus. It is the ability to focus inward instead of worrying about external stimuli. It is taking care of business.

When Your Event Begins

STRATEGIES FOR COMPETITION

1. Focus on your immediate plan: Just think about the first part of your event, take things one step at a time. When I did the RAAM, I focused on crossing one state at a time. Thinking about traversing the entire continent would have been daunting.

2. Be in the moment. Stay mindful of the present. It is too easy to let past and future fears cloud your present reality.

3. Be process-oriented. Think about your breathing, posture, or focus. Do not worry about the outcome.

4. Mentally scan your body. Are you relaxed? Is your form perfect?

5. Associate or dissociate. Check you comfort level, if you are uncomfortable, change your posture, stride length, or form. If your movement is correct, and you can afford a few moments, dissociate.

6. Take advantage. Although circumstances will not always turn out in your favor, minimize mistakes and maximize good fortune.

7. Visualize. Use imagery to see, feel, and experience yourself as strong and powerful. Perform effortlessly.

8. Minimize distractions. Let distractions go in one ear and out the other. Focus on your present effort only.

9. Talk nicely. It is human to be negative. Challenge yourself to remain positive throughout your entire event no matter what happens.

HANDLING DISCOMFORT: A PREREQUISITE FOR GREAT PERFORMANCE

Know yourself. Increase your awareness of your balance and equilibrium systems. Get in touch with your physical systems to change the maladaptive patterns that accompany pain. If you can be mindful of the physiological interactions that occur beneath your skin, you will be more adept at heading off potential injury and pain.

Your life is a training ground for mind/body. In my case:

- Karate taught me to deal with acute pain.
- Cycling taught me to deal with chronic pain.
- Tennis taught me to deal with psychological pain.

MARTIAL ARTS IMAGERY — GETTING TO THE NEXT LEVEL

As you progress, you need to continually refine your mind/body training. Search yourself to determine weakness in your mindfulness and concentration. Know that your strengths and weaknesses change depending on your circumstances and the internal manifestation of your mindfulness. If you look past your failures and ignore them, you will never improve.

Although you are looking at this page, nobody knows what is going on in your mind. You could be contemplating your next meal or mentally preparing for your martial arts workout. The same is true with physical activity. Nobody really knows what is going on in your head when you are performing *kata* or sparring. Sports commentators suggest they know what you are thinking, but do they? If you are about to win your bout, are you ecstatic or mindful of the moment? When you feel depressed or dejected, do you show your opponent, or do you wear a mask of confidence?

To understand yourself more fully and to improve your performance, try the following techniques. Be mindful of your thoughts and feelings as you go through each phase:

STRATEGIES FOR IMPROVING YOUR PERFORMANCE

- ► Think back to a performance that you would prefer to forget. Try to remember how you felt. Were you nervous? Were you distracted? Were you simply overmatched? Try to recall as much as you possibly can about yourself, your surroundings, and your feelings.

- ► Think back to a peak performance. Remember how you felt. Were you confident? Were you focused? Did you simply overwhelm your competition? Try to recall as much as possible about yourself, your surroundings, and your feelings.

- ► Compare the two. Did you notice any patterns within or between your negative and positive performances?

Practice this strategy once every six months. Just by becoming mindful of your thought processes and feelings, you will benefit your upcoming performances.

Body Language

Body language communicates volumes, without speaking a word. Pay attention to the natural tendencies of your opponent. Does he bounce lightly on his feet or remain still? Is he relaxed or tense? Is she angry or passive? Is she tentative or having fun?

If your rival is poised to defend, he or she may strike when you least expect it. Recognize cues to determine your rival's level of readiness and vulnerability. Experience teaches these signals over time; however, you can accelerate this process by learning to interpret your opponent's body language. Examine every move objectively, including gestures, eye contact, posture, hand movements, and body movements like moving forward and backward at different angles and speeds. Analyze all of them. Use them. Mindfulness will help you to objectively evaluate your opponent's every move. In time you will know what to expect.

Now turn inward and pay attention to your actions. Rather than forcing your counterattacks, relax. Do not try too hard. Redirect your opponent's attack. Be gentle but precise; brutality is unnecessary. "Weakness prevails over strength, gentleness conquers, the calm and restful breeze tames the violent sea," states Lao Tzu.

Mindfulness will teach you to control your instinctive tendencies. You are not required to actually fight or flight; simply acknowledge your inborn reactions. Know them, understand them, and counteract them if necessary. This requires discipline and mindfulness.

The fight-or-flight response is unnecessary if an opponent is aggressive. If your rival is focusing only on an attack that he or she cannot defend, allow your rival to reel you in. Then counterattack at will. Expect a physical response; your opponent will react to your attack. You take control and dictate the game. Remain one move ahead.

You can keep your opponent off guard by moving him or her around. Show your opponent something different, especially if he or she is poised to attack. Ignite his or her fight-or-flight response. Alarm will cause your opponent's body to tense. Rigid muscles cannot effectively respond to an attack. By short-circuiting his or her counterattack, you are inhibiting his or her mindfulness. If you speak your body language well enough, your opponent must respond to it. Entice your opponent by leaving an opening. Play chess. If you cannot read your opponent, wait. Patience is key. When your opponent takes the bait, jump at the opportunity and strike.

As a martial artist you spent years practicing your art, hundreds of hours of practicing and training. Expand your talents and separate yourself. Anyone can execute a throw or step; find something that is uniquely yours. Develop a special technique—a move, a fake, or a hit or kick—something that you can rely on. Put yourself into it, and determine when, why, what speed, and from what distance your technique works best. Each time you execute it, do so as if your opponent is seeing it for the first time. Make it yours.

Allow your opponent to believe he is in control. Let your rival find her comfort zone, then disarm her. If you are in control, you can guide your opponent to respond appropriately to your every move. Lead him or her in the direction of your attack. Use body language to help your opponent overlook your special technique. Then make your move. Go for it. Your opponent will not expect the power of your special technique. Let it be the final blow. Score.

Mastery is all about remaining calm and mindful. Use your brain as well as your brawn. Mindfulness will work on your toughest opponents. You may not believe the benefits of it until you try it. Casual observers cannot understand. You have nothing to lose and everything to gain. Go for it.

Motivation

Do you ever wonder why great things happen to some people and not others? Do you ever read about people who have tried this or that technique and had some incredible result, but when you try it, you do not get the same result? Have you become a person for whom nothing seems to work?

Take a look at what you have done so far in your life to get you where you are. Was it hard work or a technique based on a recommendation, or some other reason? Perhaps each time you try something new you think, "Well, it did not work that time, I will try something else." Everything else you try is compared to that first experience. You begin comparing and not really trying anything on its own merit. When you do so, you sabotage yourself. You may not automatically expect failure, but you have it as an option and perhaps even as a probability based on your previous experiences.

The more you reinforce this mindset the more you will continue do it. To combat this, stop comparing your efforts and performances with others. Do not set expectations based on someone else's results. Believe that you deserve to achieve, and you will. After you achieve, you will succeed and your life will change for the better. Do this at your own pace without preconceived notions or expectations. It will happen if you let it.

If you want to grow beyond your limitations, you need to know yourself better than anyone else does. Learn to be flexible and to adapt to any situation. Try the following exercises to help you in this endeavor.

> ► Make a list of three things you do automatically, then make a conscious decision to change them. For example, the next time you put on your pants, put your other leg in first. Change the channel without using your remote control. Try brushing your teeth with your other hand. This teaches you that if you can change the little things, you can change the big things too.
> ► Think about all of your great performances throughout the day, rather than focusing on the negative. Enjoy your accomplishments.

Tennis, cycling, and karate competitions are microcosms of my daily life. The lessons I learned from sports readily transfers to mindfulness in the real world. Remaining patient to return a serve while playing tennis and developing a killer instinct in karate competitions have helped me to attain mindfulness from the classroom to the boardroom. All of this comes from experience.

As I was racing across America, I experienced moments of ecstasy and, moments later, depression. The doldrums of surviving the desert followed by harrowing mountainous descents left me shell-shocked. Ten years later, during idle moments I flashback to my joyful pedal stroke and then recalled the pain. Everything hurt: my hands, feet, butt—any part of my body that made contact with the bike. My point is when you are presented with a seemingly insurmountable challenge, take it. You will learn more about yourself than you could have dreamed.

MUSIC

Music motivates! Though the beat is different for everyone, find your beat and use it to improve your martial arts workout. The beat can be chaotic, staccato, lyrical or still and can fuel your training.

A chaotic beat surges and darts. It carries you away like being out of control. Let your brain go and follow the music. Do not think and do not let doubts or inhibitions interfere. Just let it happen.

A staccato beat is powerful and crisp. It is hard driving and pulsating. Let the beat take over. You can focus your breathing with it, inhale and exhale to the beat.

A lyrical beat is light, bouncy, airy, playful, and exhilarating. If you combine staccato and flowing, you get lyrical.

A still rhythm provides you with an inner calm. It allows you to go within yourself. Feel emptiness and fullness. Focus on the gaps between the beat.

As you train, focus on the beat and let it overtake you in waves. Center the beat in your belly, and connect your breath to the rhythm of the music. Relax and find your natural movement, and move when your body feels like it.

Winning with Mindfulness

You can always come out on top if you show your opponent you cannot be affected. One evening, I arrived home after class and was parking my car when another car pulled up behind me. The driver jumped out and walked quickly towards me asking, "Are you the guy that cut me off back there?" Before I had a chance to speak, he pulled a knife. In doing so his comb fell to the concrete. When he reached down to retrieve it, I knew I had him. I could have kicked him in the head, and the conflict would have been resolved. Instead, when he stood up I asked, "Are you going to use that knife on me?" He looked me straight in the eye. I did not flinch. He studied me and said, "No man, I am just looking for some girls." He walked into another apartment building. In this instant I showed my would-be opponent that even his knife did not affect me—and I came out the winner.

Knowledge is a powerful ally. Become a student of your art. Become an expert. In combat, for example, there is punching, striking, grappling, grabbing, holding, and submissions. In tennis, there are serves, volleys, overheads, dropshots, and ground-strokes. In cycling, there are sitting climbs, standing climbs, sprinting, aerodynamics, and spinning.

The more you learn about your martial art, the fewer surprises you will find along the way.

Knowing your martial art can help you find meaning in everything. Training is a microcosm of your life. Through learning and practice, you become mindful. You also develop a calm and concentrated mind.

Mindfulness, perseverance, and endurance are hallmarks of success. To be your mind/body best, develop these qualities. You may even surpass someone of greater talent if you develop these inner qualities.

Physical training enhances your mindfulness. Once you are truly mindful, you no longer need to obsess about your game. Pedaling a bike, punching and kicking, or swinging a tennis racket is fun but unnecessary when you grasp the concept of mindfulness. After training in a sport or activity for ten years or more, you become your activity. Although I have not ridden my bicycle in months, if someone asked me to ride one hundred miles, I could do it. I know I could do it in less than six hours without a break and with little pain.

Hours of practicing your sport or activity will improve your creativity as well. While shadowboxing in airports, I developed new attacks, defenses, and movements. Learn the essence of your sport. Become your sport. Eat, sleep and drink your sport. Without this, you have a shallow understanding. You must continue to learn, to practice, to ponder, and create.

Eventually you will develop moves to create your own art. This happens when you have mastered your art. After twenty years of training, you may be an expert. At this point your moves are second nature. It does not matter what art you have chosen; years of mindful training have prepared you to execute awesome techniques, especially if you have competed. Others may think you are a natural, but you know work and experience placed you in the forefront.

Everything you do affects your success. Be mindful of your eating, sleeping, goal setting, discipline, physical training, and mental focus. Your art becomes your science, and you are the student.

TAME YOUR BRAIN

Tournament competitors are usually interested in learning about their opponents before locking horns. Some, however, lack concern about their upcoming matches. They try to relax without a plan of attack. They have no expectations. Without anticipation of their bouts, there is less pressure—so they choose to not know their adversary. Rather than face their fears, they prefer ignorance.

You would not build a house without a blueprint. It just does not make sense to step into the ring without tactics. Matches last only a few minutes or seconds. After the bell signals the start of the round, you have little time to prepare. It may be hard to respond if you have no game plan.

Scout your competition. Instead of worrying about your opponent's reputation, prepare by analyzing his or her technique. Elite athletes rely on a variety of cues to win. The more information at your command the better. Discuss strategies with previous competitors. Accept guidance from friends, coaches, and other fighters, and rely on your instincts.

It is better to conceive your own strategy than to use someone else's. My instructor (Sensei) from Okinawa, visited Mississippi in the mid seventies. He was surprised to see me in the finals of the State Karate Championships. During the final bout my sensei tried to coach me. However, I fought differently than when we practiced overseas. In Okinawa, our kicks were low and hard. After returning to the United States, I preferred to throw double-kicks to the head. I tried Sensei's advice to block and counterattack with low, hard kicks. His suggestions might have worked—if he was in the ring.

If you enter a match without a battle strategy you are setting yourself up for frustration. My first full-contact fight took place in Plano, Texas. My opponent (also his first full-contact fight) and I were both extremely nervous. Ed Daniels, my trainer, was a legend in the Professional Karate Association (PKA). I followed every bit of his advice, but I should have declined his decision to spread heat balm all over my body to warm me up. I was on fire. I attacked so vigorously I forgot the fight was scheduled for five rounds. Fortunately so did my opponent. Rounds two through five turned into a waltz, neither of us having the energy to raise a hand or foot. Instead of pacing ourselves, we expended all of our energy up front. The heat balm had me so fired up any plans that I had were abandoned.

If you have never seen your opponent, and you have no information about him or her, begin the match with techniques with which you are comfortable. Do not try radical, unfamiliar, or difficult movements. Analyze how your opponent reacts. Throw kicks as if playing chess. Study his responses to your aggression. Does he counterattack? Is she a technician or a brawler? Take your time, and do not judge prematurely. If your opponent blocks your best attack, that does not indicate invincibility.

Sometimes a thorough investigation of your dark horse opponent may uncover little evidence about his or her fighting style. It is extremely difficult to assess a phantom opponent. Your best assessment should come early in the match.

After your match, scrawl a page in your notebook about your opponent. Review his or her abilities and how you contended with him or her. Scribble tips that will help you for your next meeting. If you encounter this opponent a second time, beware. He or she may have improved. Just because this opponent could not block your sidekick does not mean he or she has not learned.

I once received a phone call from a buddy asking if I wanted a PKA fight on ESPN. I said, "Sure, when?" He said, "Sorry about such short notice, but it is next week." I thought a moment. I said, "Okay, but who do I fight?" He did not know. My opponent never showed for the weigh-in. The first time I laid eyes on him was in the ring. He was six-foot-four-inches, two hundred and fifty three pounds! During the introduction, I learned he played professional football for the Tampa Bay Buccaneers. I had just seconds to figure him out. My only chance was to kick and run. I did. It worked because I was able to access the situation and quickly formulate some sort of strategy. I was able to do this because I was in control of myself, and I had a lot of experience under my belt. I do not recommend that you try this, especially in the beginning.

Your Journey Begins

Success is measured in achievement. Reaching lofty goals may seem easy, that is until we peer behind the scenes. Consider Olympians, World Champions, and professional athletes. Because they make their sport look easy we sometimes forget how hard they work. Though they reap tremendous rewards you need to consider just what kind of toll they pay.

You, too, have the opportunity to experience success beyond your wildest expectations, and you can enjoy the process. However, first you must prepare. Step one is to pay attention. Which aspects of mindfulness do you enjoy? Close your eyes and take a few moments to determine your desires. Do not hesitate to explore seemingly unattainable ideals, but realize that you need to do it one step at a time. Make a detailed wish list. Nothing is far-fetched. Fantasize for hours, days, months. Know inside that it takes as long as it takes. Make mental notes or write them down. How would it feel to be competing in the World Championships? Attain mastery with your heart and mind. Feel victorious from the tips of your toes to the top of your head.

Next, set achievable short-term goals that will equip you to tackle your mission. This requires research. A fledgling competitive swimmer locates a YMCA. A novice martial artist sets aside hours for physical training. Early achievements serve as motivation, and daily short-term targets inspire you. Small successes provide endurance for the long haul.

Keep in mind that no worthwhile goal is simple. Prepare for distractions and obstacles. Motivation waxes and wanes; know that there will be pitfalls. Stay mindful and focused and be careful of those who sabotage your efforts. Part of your duties may be unrelated to your chosen dream. You may embrace competition but detest hours of training. Sometimes you are required to bide your time when you prefer to fight.

Mindfulness is sometimes perceived as one-dimensional. Keep your options open. Strive to be well rounded. Have it all, but guard your priorities. Make mindful daily choices based on your priorities and your mission. Choose training that motivates you rather than vegetating through a mindless workout. Fall asleep at a reasonable hour and wake early to prepare your day. Each hour brings you closer to health, fitness, and mindfulness.

You should not let winning or losing affect your progress. If you are disappointed with an outcome, search to discover how you may improve your performance. Competition provides you with the information so that you can be better next time if you remain mindful. Constructive criticism provides insight; do not let your ego get in the way. Improvement does not come fast or easy. Sometimes a breakthrough takes years of disciplined training. Let go and relax. If you try too hard you will undermine your efforts. Ask yourself, "Why am I training?" Think about the reasons you started in the first place.

Opportunities that take you to the next level are scarce. Be mindful for a break. Read books and magazines. Write letters to establish rapport with possible teammates. Keep an eye out for programs that relate to your dream. You may receive a phone call for a once in a lifetime bout or a master may mysteriously find you. Although the everyday grind can wear you down, pay attention to these magic moments.

Success does not just come from being better than your opponent. Success is what you do outside of your striving that counts as well. There are thousands who reach their summit and would gladly trade it for a simpler life. Self-gratification and high achievement alone are not the answer. Rather than treading on folks, carry them. Give yourself permission to be your best, yet help your comrades along the way. Unless you support your friends, you may find emptiness at the top. It is not just about winning and losing and reaching your potential. Anybody can struggle to become a champion, but how many mindfully help others become champions as well?

PRIORITIES

When you are preparing for a martial arts competition there is much to do. Physical and mental conditioning is only half the battle. The other half is politics, sponsors, and recovery. Time management becomes a priority and balance is very important. Top competitors develop mindfulness. They are able to balance training and families. Surveys of national level competitors demonstrated that sanctity was their catalyst.

You may train for health, fitness, friendships, fun, or competition. Train with those who are like-minded. If you can identify the reasons you work out with others, motivation will come easy. If you choose to compete, do it because you love it. Some people punch and kick for pleasure. Others like to spar without a referee or a stopwatch. Ask yourself, "Would I train and compete without a care of winning?" This is mindful training.

If you were an elite athlete in your youth, resist the temptation to compare your performance with others. To reach your highest levels, compete with yourself. However, most important is your attitude toward your performance. If you are mindful, your goals are constantly being refined according to your opportunities and obstacles. You alone have the power to determine your attitude.

Compete against yourself. The adulation and awards you received in high school or college stirred you, but it is equally fulfilling to perform a perfect kick. It takes perseverance and discipline to awaken early and train just for the sake of training. There will be no crowds, but you can conjure up the same excitement you experienced when you were a young competitor.

Part of the exhilaration you experienced in school was pushing your limit. You are not in that situation any longer. Ease into your conditioning until you can progressively increase your intensity. Start easy, then stretch. At first, breathe from your nose. Continue practicing. Feel the blood surging into your legs. Your breathing and heart rate speed up. Think about your form. Maintain perfect posture. Keep your upper body relaxed. Breathe deeply from your diaphragm. Feel the blood transporting oxygen to your working muscles. The lactic acid burn is intense, but work through it. When your concentration disengages, bring it back. Focus. Remain mindful.

DISCIPLINE

In today's fast lifestyle, instructors and training partners are in demand—and for good reasons: Your instructor motivates you to get out three more gut-busting repetitions. Your training partner can save your back on a heavy squat. They psyche you up and give you inspiration when you feel weak and tired. A partner also occasionally serves as a crutch to force you to work when you would rather be a couch potato.

It does not matter if you have the best instructor or most reliable workout partner; you will not get far if you lack self-discipline. Teamwork is fine, but you have got to be self-motivated if you are going to be your best. The search for improvement starts from within. Disciplined training is your path to mindfulness.

Elite players discipline both their bodies and minds. In many styles, there are no time-outs, substitutions, or coaching to give you a breather. You may be required to spend hours alone with your thoughts. Periodically examine your choices. Determine if you are struggling to reach someone else's goal. Search yourself to discover the reasons you do what you do.

Look back on your life. List your accomplishments. Any worthwhile achievement requires perseverance. Finishing school, playing a musical instrument, or hauling hay demands discipline. Draw upon your past challenges to shape your future. You already have a foundation. If you develop discipline in one thing, you can train yourself for many things.

When your mind is ready your body will follow. Lao Tsu said, "Building your body can be achieved only when your mind has been disciplined." Get hooked on disciplined training because an afternoon of lounging cannot beat a spirited workout. Some people crave alcohol or gambling, but physical training is better than any drug.

The secret is to convince yourself that martial arts is play. It is fun if you know when to start and finish. Set guidelines as to how much time to devote to training. Disciplined training requires you to set aside just a few minutes each day. Maintain your program until it is routine. Always look forward to your activity. By making it enjoyable, you avoid burn out. If priorities conflict, be flexible. Once training is a habit, it is easy.

Begin with baby steps and progress gradually. In six months, you will become accustomed to your training program. Then you can gradually increase your intensity no more than five percent for a given workout. If you are too vigorous your body will revolt. If you plan properly, however, you can discipline yourself to do almost anything.

SCHEDULE

Effective martial arts training comes from realistic goals. Be realistic about how much time you can devote to your practice. Make a schedule, allocate minutes, hours, days, weeks, or months to hone your strengths and fortify your weaknesses. Initially you may be chagrined to discover that you do not have enough time to practice and train. This is where your modifications begin by either redefining your goals or adjusting your schedule.

Once you have your strengths and weaknesses defined, you can improve them through a series of drills or exercises. This is true of both mind and body skills. In fact, while your body is resting, your mind can propel you forward using visualization, mindfulness, or focus training.

As your training continues, make changes depending on your progress. Adjust your schedule according to your skill level changes. Take time to readjust. Keep a written record of your training, schedules, and evaluations. When you succeed or fail, revisit your training program and change it. Write down your thoughts and feelings along with your physical progress. This will help you remain mindful.

STRETCH YOUR BODY AND SOOTHE YOUR MIND

Your martial arts training should extend into every aspect of your life. If you find yourself reading this book in the same position for long periods, try stretching to get your blood flowing. Stretch your lower back (quadratus laborum, erector spinae) by leaning forward in your chair, using your arms for support, and place your chest on your thighs. Then press yourself into an upright position and pull your shoulders back (scapular retraction) to stretch your chest (pectorals). Stretch the sides of your trunk (obliques) by twisting slowly to one side and then the other. Rest your ankle on your thigh into a figure-four position and lean your chest toward your knee, stretching your hip (gluteus and piriformis). Switch legs and repeat. Raise one arm above your head and place the other hand on your hip. Lean sideways until you feel a stretch in your waist. Switch hands and repeat. Grab your right elbow with your left hand, and pull it as high as you can stretching the back of your arm (triceps) and upper back (latissimus dorsi). Switch arms and repeat. Stretch your neck and trapezius muscles by bringing your chin to your chest. Then slowly look toward the ceiling. Bring your right ear toward your right shoulder and your left ear toward your left shoulder.

Do not be afraid to evaluate yourself. You can only make changes if you are truthful. Stand barefoot facing a mirror and look at yourself. How is your weight distributed? Are your feet angled? Are your hips even? Are your shoulders level and parallel with your hips? Do your toes and kneecaps face forward? Do you see the sides or back of your hands? A martial artists body should be balanced. Stretch and strengthen your body to develop symmetry.

STRENGTHENING YOUR CORE

Stand up and place your hands around your waist. Move in any direction. You will not have to move far before you feel your abdominal muscles brace.

Your midsection is the core of your movements. You can train your abdominal muscles with crunches or practice contracting them during your normal, upright posture. Why? Because most of your activities are performed while standing and strong abdominal muscles will hold you in correct posture. Electromyography studies have demonstrated that your obliques (side of your stomach muscles) are active when you are standing in any position. Improve the balance and strength in your trunk. Build your back and abdominal muscles from the inside out and train your core for internal stability.

The safest position for your low back is a neutral spine. A neutral spine simply means that you have a slight curve in your lower back. A neutral spine places the least amount of pressure on your disks, ligaments, and bones and allows you to absorb impact better. The breadth of your lordotic curve is individual, like a fingerprint. Excessive arching and flattening of your back stresses your spinal disks. This leads to nerve root irritation, degeneration of the vertebrae and herniated discs. Chronic pain may be caused by gravity pulling you out of alignment while you are sitting or standing. Be mindful of your posture at all times.

Develop a strong midsection, but not at the expense of a painful back. Crunches performed with a flat back are effective, but return to neutral after each repetition to maintain functional stability. As you practice your crunches, be mindful of your spine. In minutes, gravity and lack of mindfulness can pull you out of your perfect alignment. It takes practice and muscular endurance to stay in a neutral spine position. Try spending five minutes at a time in neutral position. Each week add two minutes until you can mindfully sit through your favorite sitcom in neutral spinal alignment.

Be mindful of your neutral spine while sitting, standing, and exercising. Even when you are reading, be aware of your posture and adjust your spine into pelvic neutrality. Notice how healthy it feels to release unwanted tension.

Your torso is the connection between your upper and lower limbs. A synergy between body parts will provide stability for your training. Acute back injuries occur from failing to stabilize your torso. A powerful core allows you to move with less likelihood of injury.

Mindful Martial Arts Training

BEFORE YOU BEGIN

Imagine your martial arts workout. Sport psychology studies show that if you think about throwing a punch or kick, you can actually enhance the nerve-to-muscle function, so that when you actually throw your punches and kicks, they will be faster, higher and more powerful.

Visualize your techniques as clearly as you can. Always visualize that you are executing with perfect form. Use as many senses as possible. Allow your imaginary punches and kicks to flow. In your mind "Feel" your punches and kicks extend and retract as if you were actually performing your workout. When you have completed your last imaginary kick, feel refreshed, alert, and ready to begin.

MINI-WORKOUTS

Martial arts can be practiced in a gym, hotel room, bus station, airport, or just about anywhere you can find room. Stay within yourself. Don't worry that others may be watching.

Mini-martial arts workouts (ten to twenty minutes long) are short but intense. Begin with a slow shadowboxing warmup, followed by thirty seconds of easy stretching. Then blast into high speed punches and low kicks. Gradually, increase the intensity of your kicks until within five minutes you are kicking easily to head level. Explode against your imaginary opponent with fervor.

Within minutes, punch and kick fast, high and with power. Since each martial arts workout is very short, it is easy to give one hundred percent. During the last two minutes of each mini-workout, cool down by gradually bringing your kicks down to waist and knee level. Finish with some light stretching. These mini-martial arts training sessions are truly invigorating.

MIND/BODY MARTIAL WORKOUT SUGGESTIONS

A mirror provides you with immediate feedback about your punching and kicking form, speed and intensity. Begin with an easy warmup. Then perform slow-motion strength-kicks. Follow them with punch-kick combinations. During combinations, scrutinize your form in the mirror. Is your back straight? Did you telegraph the kick? Would it have worked in a fighting situation? After about twenty minutes of combinations, cool down and stretch. This is your time to prepare yourself to re-enter the real world.

WORKOUT NO MATTER WHAT

For a change of pace, shadowbox. Let your mind wander. Dissociate. Let your attention drift. Or, think about an unsolved problem. Who knows, you may come up with a solution. Although dissociation is a nice change of pace, don't make it a habit. It is a "lazy" form of meditation.

There will be times when you're not in the mood to train, but you know you should. Drink some water. If you haven't eaten in a couple of hours, have a snack. Then convince yourself to warm up. If you don't feel like completing your entire martial arts workout, that's okay, but at least warm up. After your warmup, if you're still tired, call it a day. Nine times out of ten, your warmup will inspire you to complete your martial arts workout.

To flow from one technique to the next more smoothly, and to perform multiple combinations with ease, try these strategies:

STRATEGIES FOR LINKING MOVEMENTS

---

1. Remain relaxed. When you try too hard, you tense your muscles.

2. Focus on one thing at a time such as bent knee, speed, timing, angle of foot or target area. Trying to think about more than one item at a time will confuse your coordination.

3. Slow down. If you try to move too fast when a technique is not well learned, it will appear jerky.

4. Compete only against yourself. If you are training with others, punch and kick at your pace. not theirs. This is your workout.

Martial arts agility and balance may be improved by practicing the following drills:

STRATEGIES FOR AGILITY AND BALANCE

1. Always keep your supporting knee slightly bent on all kicks.

2. Practice slow punches and kicks with your eyes closed.

3. Attempt to throw more than a single kick consecutively (for example, double roundhouse kicks with the same leg) while remaining balanced on your other leg.

4. Practice throwing your kicks in slow motion so that your stabilizer muscles must work overtime to maintain balance.

To throw your techniques with focus and purpose, try the following:

STRATEGIES FOR PURPOSE AND FOCUS

1. Imagine attacking an opponent every time you punch and kick.

2. Strike an imaginary opponent with the correct contact surface (for instance, first two knuckles for a punch).

3. Focus your eyes on the solar plexus of your imaginary opponent.

4. Relax. Contract your muscles only at the completion of your punch or kick. This increases the speed, force and power of your technique.

MODELING

One way to try and understand what it is like to spend time in the ring is to pay attention to professional boxers and kickboxers. Watch them fight. Notice their relaxed countenance. Observe how they carry themselves. If you are viewing them on television, get off of your easy chair and follow along. Punch, kick, and block. Imagine blocking their kicks. Slip their punches. Then practice in a mirror. Model your favorite fighters. Make their techniques your own. Rather than staring without blinking, relax your gaze. Focus on your imaginary opponent, without allowing your eyes to telegraph your intentions.

TROUBLESHOOTING COMMON MISTAKES

The most common mistakes I have witnessed in martial arts training are:

TRAINING STRATEGIES

1. Warming up too fast.

2. Forgetting to stretch.

3. Letting your elbows telegraph your punches by flinging them away from your body prior to extension.

4. Muscling your punches. That is, pushing your punches instead of throwing them.

5. Throwing high-intensity combinations early in the workout.

6. Hyperextending elbows and knees.

7. Attempting to kick too high, causing your spine to go out of neutral alignment.

8. Throwing more than ten consecutive unilateral kicks.

9. Kicking to your intended imaginary opponent with the wrong part of your foot.

10. Allowing your recovery period to be too short between high-intensity intervals.

11. Failure to retract your punch or kick at the same trajectory, and at the same speed, that you extended it.

In the first few months of training, perfect your punching and kicking form. Your primary training aid should be a mirror. Later, you may decide to add intensity by punching and kicking a bag or target pad. These devices allow you to add speed and power to all of your techniques.

However, if your wrists are not firm and your toes are not pulled back you will feel it, and possibly injure yourself. So at first, hit softly, and like always, gradually progress to increased power.

BAG WORK

Warm up before striking the bag. Begin slowly! Relax and focus. Maintain proper form. Launch your movements from the ground up. When you punch, use hand wraps and bag gloves. Make sure that the point of impact for punches is your first two knuckles. For kicks, make contact with the top of your foot, the ball of your foot, your heel, or the side of your foot.

At first, perform single techniques. After you have practiced jabs, reverse punches, hooks, front kicks, roundhouse kicks, and side kicks, perform your combinations exactly as you would use them in martial arts. Keep your hands up, stay light on your feet, and imagine the bag as your opponent. Cool down by slowly shadowboxing the bag. Conclude with stretching.

TARGET PAD TRAINING

Target pads can help sharpen your punches and kicks. Be sure to warm up and stretch before using them. Go slowly at first. Touch the pad with each strike. After a thorough warmup, snap your kicks and punches, but not too hard. Remember never to fully extend your knees. Retract your foot as quickly as you threw it. Hit with the appropriate part of your foot.

Your partner can hold a pad in each hand, providing you with moving targets. (Be sure never to hold the pads in front of your face, for obvious reasons.) Each time your partner moves the pads, execute a different kick or punch. For example, if the target is facing down, do a front kick. If it is down at a forty-five degree angle, throw a roundhouse kick. If it is perpendicular to the floor, shoot a side kick. Throw your punches and kicks from your fighting position. Watch your partner's solar plexus and see the pads peripherally. Punch and kick with perfect form and enjoy the feeling of contact.

Other Mind/Body Workouts

MINDFUL STATIONARY CYCLING

Your stationary bike is a tool. It is a piece of metal designed to help you achieve physical fitness and mindfulness. Pedaling is more than just turning little circles with your feet. You need to be relaxed and focused on your bike. Breathe correctly, and concentrate on perfect form. Talk to yourself in a positive way, visualize your pedal stroke, and associate it with your muscles.

When you pedal a stationary bike, you promote the relaxation your body requires. Fast spinning will stress to your body whereas pedaling at a relaxed cadence produces profound relaxation. The practice of mind/body cycling drills allows you to experience a continuum of extremes in a controlled setting.

Pedaling an exercise bike for twenty minutes can reduce stress, but mind/body cycling will goes a step further. Mind/body strategies such as imagery and association provide you with mindfulness that will transfer to your life off the bike. Mindfulness helps you relax. As you exercise on the bike, practice deep-breathing and tension-releasing exercises; use them to help alleviate the stresses you face in the real world.

It is important to relax before, during, and after your ride. Warm up and cool down with a relaxed attitude. Enjoy muscle relaxation throughout your workout. I do not mean a wet noodle type of relaxation, but the kind of relaxation that allows you to be alert and focused with each pedal stroke. The following technique may help you relax as you train.

While in a seated position on the bike, pedal gently and relax. Breathe from your diaphragm, keep your shoulders back and down, and be sure that your lower back maintains a natural arch in neutral spinal alignment. Relax your entire body but do not force it. Become especially aware of upper body tension and let those muscles relax. Allow tension to be released. Relaxation will happen if you clear your mind and glide through your pedal stroke. When your legs relax, pedal automatically, easily, and efficiently. As you pedal focus on your breath. Take deep breaths inhaling through your nose and exhaling through pursed lips. Inhale through your nose for four pedal strokes to expand your lungs. As you do this, breathe from your diaphragm instead of your chest. Focus on raising your diaphragm. Fill your lower, central, and upper chest, in that order. Then take eight pedal strokes to exhale through pursed lips while lowering your diaphragm.

Combine mindfulness with deep breathing and pedaling. Take deep breaths from your diaphragm with long exhalations. When you breathe from your navel, your diaphragm is activated. This allows you to take deeper, longer breaths, using more of your lung capacity. Double-time your pedal stroke, your breathing and heart rate will increase. Continue to breathe deeply from your diaphragm so your stomach pushes out. Take in as much oxygen as possible. Imagine oxygen-filled blood cells nourishing your legs. Exhale automatically. Your pedals will fly on their own accord as you practice mindfulness. The more you do it, the easier it will become to focus on your breath.

Pedaling is unique to you and your fitness needs and goals. You are in control of the resistance and the speed. Decide when to challenge your body and when to relax. Immerse yourself in your pedaling. Try to pedal and relax simultaneously, use your pedal stroke as your mantra. Each rhythmic revolution will relax your mind and body. Mindfulness is not difficult or time consuming, but simply a matter of focusing on each pedal stroke. Let distractions pass through your mind. Pedal and breathe at your individual cadence. Personalize it. The timing is yours, not an instructor's; there is no competition. Once you decide the level at which to perform, let nothing distract or disturb you, just pedal and breathe.

As you pedal in the moment, monitor the mechanics of your pedal stroke. Be sure the knees are over your toes. Your movements should be piston-like. Do not mash the pedals. Mashing occurs when you press too hard on the pedals, and sometimes leads to knee and hip problems. Challenge yourself. Stand and pull from your hamstrings on the upstroke. This will introduce new stresses to your workout.

Psychologists claim humans need some stress/discomfort in order to function. We seek an optimum level of discomfort—a level we can handle. It is common, that when confronted with fatigue, the first option is to quit. Mindfulness can help you get through this. If your goal is to succeed, it is useful to persevere. Expect to get through discomfort. Mindfulness allows you to relax, and relaxation is a potent painkiller. When I rode 458 miles in a 24-hour ultra-marathon cycling race, I experienced pain the entire time. Rather than succumb, I acknowledged the pain's presence and focused on my rock-and-roll audiotape. Remaining mindful of the music was my painkiller. Pain is an in-the-moment experience. Pain protects you from injury. While experiencing the doldrums of the Race Across America, I promised I would never do ultra-distance cycling again. A week after completing the race, however, I was training for next year's event. Experiencing mindfulness for the ten-day Race Across America far outweighed the discomfort.

MINDFUL STAIR CLIMBING

Try the mindful strategy below as you are stair climbing. It can, of course, be modified for use with any rhythmic aerobic endeavor.

STRATEGIES FOR STAIR CLIMBING

1. Begin your stair climbing by selecting your program setting for manual control. Set the time for twenty minutes. Concentrate on your breathing. Breathe deeply from your diaphragm. Feel your rib cage and abdomen expand with each breath. Count your steps on each inhalation and exhalation. Focus only on the relationship between your steps and your breath.

2. Feel your feet as they press into the platform. Continue to focus on the rhythm of your breath.

3. Allow your awareness to sink into your gluteus and hips. Feel the power of each step and notice how your breath energizes each step.

4. Bring your attention to a spot a few inches below your navel. Each step begins and ends here.

5. Close your eyes. See yourself climbing each step with confidence and control.

6. Tell yourself how good you feel.

INDOOR CYCLING AND STAIR CLIMBING
FATIGUE CONTROL

As you practice these techniques you will experience various levels of fatigue. Below are phases one and two of a strategy that can be used to overcome fatigue.

STRATEGIES FOR CONTROLLING FATIGUE

Phase 1

1. Fatigue exists in your mind.

2. Know that you can beat fatigue and discomfort.

3. Go with it. Pushing yourself through discomfort will lead you to your goal.

4. Increase your pedaling or stepping speed, but expect an increase in discomfort.

5. An increase in the burn is a signal you are nearing the finish line.

6. Be objective about the burn and fatigue. Observe it. Enjoy it.

Phase 2

1. You have the power to control your thoughts.

2. Your mind can focus on only one thing at a time.

3. When the lactic acid burn or stepping fatigue become unbearable, change your focus.

4. Enjoy focusing on your beat; the discomfort will disappear.

MIND/BODY RESISTANCE TRAINING

As you have seen thus far, mind/body techniques can be utilized during any physical activity. The following strategy can be used to bring a new level to your resistance workouts.

STRATEGIES FOR IMPROVING RESISTANCE WORKOUTS

1. Review your training goals (e.g. bigger biceps, stronger bench press).

2. Begin each exercise with perfect posture and maintain it through the duration of your set.

3. Warm up with some easy repetitions as you prepare your mind/body for a perfect workout.

4. Visualize and feel the muscle group you are preparing to train. Imagine all of your muscle fibers recruited for each repetition.

5. Begin your first repetition with confidence and continue your workout until you have completed your entire program.

6. Feel great about yourself for reaching your workout goals.

STRATEGIES FOR MENTAL TOUGHNESS

1. Stay mentally pumped up even when you are physically tired.

2. Act as if you are enjoying your pedaling, climbing, or lifting, even when you are not.

3. Plan your strategy prior to each drill or set.

4. Follow the same rituals before beginning each workout.

5. The higher the intensity of your pedaling, stepping, or lifting, the more you love it.

6. Thrive on having fun while training.

7. Stay positive regardless of how much you hurt.

8. By increasing awareness of your mental strengths and weaknesses, you will be better equipped to consistently perform toward the upper range of your ability.

Mind/Body 24 Hours a Day

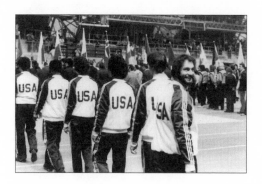

✳ Mind/Body 24 Hours a Day ✳

Eating to Fuel Your Body and Mind

Your body responds to the demands you place on it whether they are good or bad. There is eustress (good stress that drives you to succeed and fuels your hopes and dreams) and distress (bad stress that causes anxiety, illness, and depression). Handle stress mindfully and you can cope with anything.

Coping with stress requires energy so you need to fuel your body if you want it to cope successfully. Stress and nutrition are linked. If you are deficient in a certain nutrient, your body will be put in a stressful situation and respond accordingly. Anxiety, for example, interferes with your nutrient absorption and retention. If you are well nourished, you are better equipped to deal with stress.

Vitamins and minerals also play an important role as to how your immune system reacts. Your immune system is responsible for defending your body against infection and disease. When your body is stressed, it releases hormones that suppress your immune system. This exposes your body to infection. Vitamins C and B, beta carotene, and trace minerals help your immune system stay strong to fight the debilitating effects of stress.

Your diet affects your ability to cope with stress. If you cut down on refined carbohydrates, sugar, and caffeine, and you consume more whole grain breads, cereals, and other nutritious foods, you are on a stress-busting diet. Your nutrition program should include fruits, vegetables, whole grain breads and cereals, beans and peas, low-fat or non-fat dairy products, several glasses of water, and lean meats (chicken and fish).

MINDFULNESS IN YOUR EATING

We know that fad diets do not work. If you focus on foods you should not be eating, you will crave them all the more. Instead, think of wonderful combinations of lean meats, fruits, and vegetables. There are no forbidden foods, simply healthier choices. Rather than feeling deprived, enjoy energy and health on your newfound eating program. Set flexible, short-term, attainable eating goals rather than trying to lose fifty pounds and never eating ice cream again. Immediate, excessive weight loss means that you are losing it too fast—you will gain it back. A program you cannot do for the rest of your life is not worth trying for a single day. If you fall off the wagon, just get back on. It is not one meal or a day of eating that matters, it is the weeks and months of better food choices that keep you motivated to stay on your program. Rather than obsessing about food, eat several times a day to stabilize your blood sugar and fuel your exercise. Listen to your body. If you are hungry, eat. When you are satisfied, stop. It is that simple.

After your workout you may prefer to lounge, but if you do, lounge at a snack bar. Within an hour of completing your workout, eat or drink a carbohydrate/protein combination in a 4-to-1 ratio. A cup of yogurt, energy bar, protein-carbohydrate shake, or a half of a sandwich will do the trick. Your brain and muscles require carbohydrates for energy, but protein rebuilds the micro-tears that occur in your muscle tissue during your workout. You need both. This carbohydrate-protein combination following exercise also strengthens your immune system. Unlike the exerciser who falls in front of the television after a workout, you should feel invigorated after your training. Refueling your body makes sure you are fully rehydrated. Dehydration leads to fatigue and listlessness. Ironically, water alone does not always do the trick. If you work out a lot and drink water without replenishing your sodium, potassium, chloride, and magnesium, you can actually suffer from water intoxication (hyponatremia). It is important, therefore, to choose a sports drink or a variety of fruits such as bananas, oranges, tomatoes, and potatoes to keep your mind/body healthy and ready.

VITAMINS AND MINERALS

It is important to understand how vitamins and minerals keep you body balanced. The following list can provide you with a starting point of nutritional understanding.

Vitamin A. Helps to maintain good vision, prevents night blindness. It also aids in growth, repair, and maintenance of your body tissues.

Beta-Carotene. Strengthens your immune system, maintains healthy skin and eyes, prevents night blindness, and protects skin from ultraviolet rays.

Vitamin B-Complex. Belongs to a family of essential water-soluble vitamins that complement each other.

Vitamin B1 (Thiamine). Important for metabolizing carbohydrates into energy and for normal function of the nervous system.

Vitamin B2 (Riboflavin). Required for vision, growth, and absorption of iron. It is also essential for healthy skin, nails, hair, and eyes, as well as the formation of antibodies.

Vitamin B3 (Niacinamide). Essential for normal body balance and the health of the nervous system. Is involved in hundreds of biochemical reactions in the body.

Vitamin B5 (Pantothenic Acid). Essential for the synthesis of cholesterol and fatty acids and maintaining a healthy digestive tract.

Vitamin B6 (Pyridoxine HCI). Required for processing fats, carbohydrates and protein, utilizing linoleic acid and the production of antibodies and red blood cells.

Vitamin B12 (Cyanoco Balamin). Aids the normal synthesis of red blood cells and proper utilization of fats, carbohydrates, and protein.

Vitamin B15. Helps increase oxygen supply to active tissue.

Choline. Essential for the health of kidneys, liver, and arteries.

Inositol. Promotes the growth and color of hair, healthy intestinal activity, control of blood cholesterol, and healthy bone marrow and eye membranes.

PABA (Para Amino Benzoic Acid). Helps utilize protein and is important in the maintenance of healthy skin and hair. A growth factor.

Biotin. Aids in metabolizing carbohydrates and fats into energy.

Folic Acid. Essential in synthesizing DNA and RNA. Also important in protein metabolism, reproduction, growth, and the formation of red blood cells.

Vitamin C. Essential in the formation of collagen fiber in the skin, bones, and ligaments. Beneficial against bone and tooth weakness.

Vitamin D. Also known as the Sunshine Vitamin because it can be provided in part by the sun. Essential for the assimilation of calcium, the growth and development of bones, teeth, and jaw formulation, and the maintenance of blood coagulation and cardiac rhythm.

Vitamin E. Essential for the assimilation of vitamins A, C, and D. Promotes healthy heart and lungs, decreases the pain associates with childbirth, and oxygenates tissues.

Calcium. Essential for the transportation of nerve impulses, blood coagulation, vitamin C utilization, reduction of cavities, and formation of strong bones.

Iron. Vital component of hemoglobin, the oxygen carrying pigment of the red blood cells. Also essential for the production of energy and normal brain function.

Magnesium. Calms the nervous system.

Manganese. Essential for normal reproductive functions, milk formulation, building resistance to disease and activating enzymes important for carbohydrate and fat production.

Niacin. Essential for the efficient use of protein.

Potassium. Essential for balancing your system, controlling body fluids, normalizing the heartbeat, nourishing the muscles, and assisting the kidneys' disposal of body waste.

Too Busy for Mindfulness

A famous tightrope walker said, "Life is on the wire, everything else is waiting." Paying attention to relaxation and concentration is difficult when your world is filled to the max. Monks sit on mountaintops and contemplate the universe. They have time because "everyday" distractions are not an issue. Your life, however, is overflowing with distractions. Goals, relationships, hopes, dreams, and work keep you busy—not to mention the time you spend watching television, listening to the radio, and reading the newspaper.

MAKING TIME

What options do you have, other than relocating to Tibet? First, you can slice away unnecessary activities that do not allow for mindfulness. For example, limit the time you spend watching television and other nonessential activities. It is better to stare at a blank wall and achieve a thoughtless state than it is to let your brain be captured by a mindless sitcom. Be mindful of how you pursue your free time.

When you are in active pursuit of something, whether it be a vocation, activity, or hobby, do it fully. Rather than watch television while reading the paper, simply read the paper and focus on it. Prepare for and strive to achieve a goal rather than mindlessly stumble through your day. Regardless of your ultimate plan or your true potential, take the time to modulate your activation and focus your attention. This is mindfulness.

This is not an end to your fun. If you are mindful, enjoyment comes naturally. Relaxation allows for openness to change. You will experience greater joy and handle life's stress with greater ease. When your mind/body is tight, flexibility is no where in sight. In this situation, pain lasts longer and is more intense; joy is short-lived.

REMAINING MINDFUL

Medical doctors are quick to point out that psychological stress leads to physical mal-adaptation and that tension exacerbates injury. To avoid these negative effects, your goal is to remain mindful under any circumstance. If you are under the duress of a medical emergency, the pain of an acute injury, or the chronic fight-or-flight response reaction to daily stress, be mindful and handle the crisis. Sometimes insidious low-stress problems are more tedious than acute ones. It is easy to mindfully focus during an onslaught. The trick is to mindfully handle trivial, less than painful, but chronically debilitating stress.

High achievers have a hard time waiting. Especially when it appears as if others are getting ahead. Waiting is very therapeutic. A little lounging does not hurt your chances of reaching your goals. Be wary that lethargy does not become a consistent pattern, however. If it does you can become lazy. Be mindful of your mind/body choices, and do what is right for you.

Choose to use or lose every moment. If you are a compulsive doer, then sitting with no thought is not a bad idea. If you are sedentary by nature, however, productive thoughts can create powerful inertia to get you off the couch. Mindfully choose what to do, moment by moment. There are thousands of mind/body strategies you can do anytime and anywhere. Think about: breathing with focus through pursed lips, tapping your foot, blinking, and postural swaying just to name a few.

- Focused breathing through pursed lips. While sitting, control your exhalations. Contract your abdominal muscles to force small puffs of air through your pursed lips. Watch the rhythm of your breath. There is no need to control your exhalations. Instead, just relax. Sometimes exhale two short bursts instead of one. You can also take a long inhalation and exhale like rapid-fire. Vary your breathing patterns such as, exhale in three bursts and inhale with one. Play with your breath and make your own patterns.
- Foot tapping. Tap your foot to any rhythm or with no rhythm at all. Just tap. Connect your mind to your foot. Pay attention to your tapping and let your mind drift.
- Blinking. Blinking your eyes is an automatic response, but you can also control your blink rate. Try to slow your blinking. Let your eyes close and then open ever so slowly. Feel the profound activation reduction. Blinking slowly tricks your mind into thinking it is time to prepare for sleep and reduces your arousal.

FLEXIBLE THINKING AND GOAL SETTING

Choose to be flexible in your approach to mindfulness. If you are flexible, you can create a variety of options. Flexible thinking allows you to go with the flow. Relax and use your mind/body. Understand that mindfulness is with you in every endeavor. Whether you are bored, tired, anxious, or laughing, a flexible mindset allows for more productivity and more fun.

If you remain flexible, you can handle any situation regardless of its difficulty. Nothing will tear you down. If you break a situation into manageable pieces, then you can control anything. First determine what you want to accomplish. This sounds easy, but it requires some soul searching. Once your long-range goal has been determined, set a series of short-term markers. These are reality checks, and they help you re-evaluate your program and methods. Once you start this process, you can ask yourself the following questions.

- Do you have all of the ingredients you need to succeed?
- Do you need to work on some areas more than others?
- Are you psychologically strong, mentally tough and disciplined, and spirited with tenacity?

Answer these questions honestly so you can develop objectives.

Your strengths are not present in equal parts and your skills can be balanced in different proportions. For example, compensate for a lack of speed with an abundance of strength. If you have a weak offense, develop an impregnable defense. Mindfulness is a balancing act. There is always something to improve.

Enlist the aid of your sensei, coach or objective peers to sharpen your strengths and bolster your weaknesses. At this point, you know where to start and what to accomplish. You may make some modifications along the way but you have a framework to begin.

Now that you have a start and end point, set a series of goals to be achieved along the way. For example, you may hope to become an Olympian. A realistic progression of goals would include local tournaments, regional championships, national championships, Pan Am Games, World Championships, and Olympic Games. This is a series of measurable accomplishments that will gauge your progress. Along with these goals, mindfully develop a series of technical goals, such as the improvement of particular techniques to improve your performance.

Some of my martial arts students were so talented that winning came easily. They were not required to work for their goals. Victory came naturally. Those naturals, however, were enslaved by their potential. At first they enjoyed competition, but getting to the next level required work. A few trained hard to become superstars, but most gave up.

Mastery does not come easy. If you work hard you can reach the limits of your naturally-given potential. As you accumulate trophies and medals, watch yourself grow. Your mindfulness remains, while trophies and medals get lost and thrown away. The more difficult your goal, the more inner strength you build.

Taking baby steps toward your dream requires discipline, and discipline comes from within yourself. One goal will lead you to another. Each succeeding purpose becomes more important than the one previously conquered. Your passion propels you forward. Even world class martial artists must conquer the little things along the way. Worldly glory has no bearing on the discipline and perseverance required to establish inner strength. Remain mindful at all times and you will enjoy your progress.

Learn from Everyone

I travel the country most weekends presenting fitness programs. Remaining mindful of the people and surroundings I encounter is stimulating. The different in dialects as well as temperaments that I encounter during my travel is astounding. I am not speaking about my clients; I am referring, for example, to shuttle drivers that take me to and from airports and hotels. Most of them enjoy good conversation, as if they have not spoken all day. One man's grandson was the mayor of Orlando and another driver owned the van company he represented. An older Italian gentleman suggested my generation has it too easy. Several drivers were recovering alcoholics and drug addicts, and they always had great stories. I even helped a taxi driver market his patented mouthguard.

The reason I am mentioning these drivers is that many are quite intelligent and mindful people. One driver actually inspired me to write this book. He demonstrated he was no different than I. We were both in hot pursuit of the truth. It is not as if these men were speaking of abstract eternal truths; they were simply middle class folks who understood there was no benefit in wasting their lives trying to become rich. It is not that they did not value money, but they realized their time was too precious to have such a narrow focus.

What did I learn from these individuals? First, I discovered a sense of humor is a prerequisite for mindfulness. Their hardships were endured because they were hilarious. While I fretted about making my flight, they were concerned about their rent. They were mindful, I was not. They realized everything would be fine, while I continued to obsess about my flight. They were content with their day-to-day existence. Mindful individuals transform fight-or-flight anxiety into an adrenaline power rush. That is, they transformed adrenal overload into a positive outcome. These shuttle drivers live fairly relaxed lives.

You probably look forward to a comfortable life. Rather than drive a van, you might prefer to sit in an air-conditioned office or watch television all day. If you always choose ease, you miss out. Your most difficult endeavors are the rewarding ones. Although at the time it may not seem this way, difficult times make you tough and resilient. Remaining mindful enables you to endure hardship.

Whether you have the goals of a world-class martial artist or someone saving for retirement, you deal with trials and tribulations on a daily basis. You find problems to worry about and solve them. Anxiety and worry can sneak up on you no matter how tough you are. Expect angst and cope with it. Although there is no magic formula, you must choose what works for you. Depend on your mindfulness to steer you in the right direction.

You have a lot in common with sport-superstars and successful businessmen. Motivation, a willingness to succeed against the odds, and the ability to stand up after a loss are probably the most important ingredients to your progress. Giving up is not an option regardless of how bad things get. When things get rough, pause, re-evaluate, and then forge ahead. Remain mindful every step of the way, and you will make the right decisions to achieve your goal. Whether you are training for the Race Across America or for a position at a local McDonald's, it is all the same. Set your sights high. Do the best that you can. Expect everything and expect nothing. If you truly love what you do, you will find success.

Sleep

Getting only a few hours of sleep each night hinders metabolism and hormone production in a way similar to the effects of aging and the early stages of diabetes. Chronic sleep loss may speed the onset or increase the severity of age-related conditions such as type-two diabetes, high blood pressure, obesity, and memory loss. One week of sleep deprivation alters hormone levels and capacity to metabolize carbohydrates. For example, during sleep-deprivation, blood sugar levels take 40 percent longer to drop following a high-carbohydrate meal that they normally do. Lack of sleep is like adding a ton of stress to your life.

If you do not provide your body with enough rest, your mind will rebel. Once the rebellion starts your body will follow. During the Race Across America, I slept twenty minutes every six hours. I continued this strategy until I reached Colorado where I tried to make up some time by missing a sleep break. That was my biggest mistake in the race. I began to wobble uncontrollably and was required by RAAM officials to sleep. I told my support crew to wake me in an hour. They tried and tried to wake me every hour for the next four hours, but my body had adapted to my twenty-minute cycle of sleep, and I had unwittingly broke the habit. My body rebelled. I fell from eighth place to fifteenth place. If I had mindfully remained with my schedule instead of succumbing to my ego, I might have finished in eighth place.

Sometimes it takes seemingly forever to fall asleep because you cannot stop thinking about tomorrow. Your alarm wakes you but you know you are not fully awake. It is suggested that about fifty million Americans are chronically sleep deprived. It is not exactly known how much sleep each individual requires because we are all biologically different; our needs vary. Some fortunate few seem to get by on only five or six hours of sleep while others need ten hours every night. In general, most healthy adults need between seven and nine hours of quality sleep each night. You know you are not getting enough sleep if you are tired all of the time, uncharacteristically irritable, fall asleep in boring situations, or rely on caffeine to get you through the day. Become mindful of your alertness, reaction times, and temperament, and adjust your sleep patterns to balance them.

Your body has a natural tendency to slow down between 1:00 P.M. and 4:00 P.M. If your schedule allows a fifteen to twenty minute siesta during this time it would be helpful. Longer than twenty minutes, however, and you will wake up feeling groggy and you might have difficulty falling asleep that night, causing even more sleep debt. Sleep is essential to your physical and mental health. Sleep deprivation causes strength loss, impaired immune function, and increased blood pressure. The lack of sleep decreases concentration and impairs your memory, learning, logical reasoning, and your ability to make mathematical calculations.

Changing your sleep pattern cannot be accomplished overnight, but it can be done in a few weeks. If serious fatigue or chronic insomnia persists, make it a point to see your physician. A good night's sleep is as important as your diet and exercise program.

Although you may be in your bed for ten hours, you may not be getting quality sleep. If you are stressed, you may feel groggy when you awaken from a full night of lying in your bed. You can combat this, however, by taking a hot shower before bedtime. When you crawl into bed, your body temperature will drop, and you will fall into a deeper level of sleep.

The quality of your sleep affects your workouts, and your workouts affect your sleep. At the Olympic Training Center in Colorado Springs, Herb Perez, a member of the United States Taekwondo Team, was preparing for his Olympics debut. Herb confided that he could not fall asleep the night before his matches. As a sport psychologist for the medical team, I suggested Herb not worry how well he would sleep the night before his bout. What mattered was the quality of sleep he got in the months before his event. Herb went on to win a Gold Medal in the Olympic Games.

Forty million Americans have some sort of sleep problem, and one in three have difficulty falling asleep. Additionally, Americans today sleep an average of ninety minutes less than they did a century ago. Minor sleep loss can impair alertness and visual skills, but chronic sleep deprivation reduces your vigilance, mental abilities, muscle strength, and aerobic capacity. Insomnia affects your ability to handle stress and solve problems. Lack of sleep can hinder your job performance. Sleep deprivation has been related to disasters including Chernobyl and the

Exxon Valdez. How many accidents have you heard about where people have dozed at the wheel of their automobiles?

Activity helps you fall asleep quicker and improve the quality of your deep sleep. Try training during the day and keep it moderate. It may be counterproductive to experience too much exercise or to work out just before bedtime. Late afternoon activity seems to be the best time to enhance your sleep. Activity especially improves sleep for those with low fitness levels and older adults. Regardless of whether activity benefits sleep because of increased fatigue, elevated body temperature, or decreased stress, it works!

The following are tips that may help you get quality sleep.

STRATEGIES FOR QUALITY SLEEP

1. Eat a snack before bedtime. Keep it light. High fat foods require a longer period to digest. A bowl of fiber cereal or half a tuna sandwich works for me.

2. Establish a step-by-step routine. Your children have a routine—bath, book, and bed. As an adult, you still need to establish your own routines and rituals. Read, watch the news, and brush your teeth. Take a bath and enjoy a sitcom or read a novel. It does not matter what you do. Just be consistent. Your body will fall into a routine, and your brain will relax.

3. If you need to catch up on sleep, go to bed an hour early. Wake up at your normal time, even on weekends.

4. Your mattress should be firm, not hard. Shut your door, turn your telephone off, turn on your answer machine, close your eyes, and sleep. The world can do without you for a little while.

5. Try to get to sleep, and arise at a consistent time. Your body enjoys regular sleep habits.

6. If you do not fall asleep after thirty minutes of lying in bed, get up. It should take you about fifteen minutes to fall asleep. If it takes you thirty minutes, do not just lie in bed tossing and turning. Get up and do something relaxing like taking a warm bath, read a book, or listen to soft music. Drink a glass of warm milk or use your progressive relaxation or breathing strategies.

7. Use your bedroom for sleep. Do not watch television or read in bed, or your brain will think it is okay to stay awake while lying in your bed.

8. Be careful of caffeine in soft drinks and chocolate as well as in coffee too close to bedtime. Nicotine can inhibit sleep as well. Alcohol can interrupt your sleep later in the night because it becomes a stimulant after the body metabolizes it.

9. Exercising regularly can greatly improve the quality of your sleep, but do it at least three hours before bedtime. Some people may need to exercise up to six hours before bedtime in order to allow themselves enough time to unwind.

Massage

Some may interpret massage as the lazy man's way to mindfulness. It is not. It is a passive method of achieving a relaxed countenance. Rather than punch, pedal or play your way to cosmic consciousness, a massage practitioner manipulates your muscles and joints to help you find a relaxed focus. There are more than fifty different types of massage. Many are variations of each other. Most massage regimens are from one of the following large categories—European massage, Western massage, Structural/Functional/Movement integration, Asian methods, or Energetic methods (non-Asian)

EUROPEAN MASSAGE includes methods based on conventional Western strategies. Techniques utilize the manipulation of soft tissue and follow the basic rules of anatomy and physiology. Practitioners use flowing and gliding strokes, usually toward the heart, tracing the outer contours of your body. They also use strokes that lift, roll, or knead your tissue. Friction, vibration, and tapping movements are also in vogue with this type of massage.

SWEDISH MASSAGE is the most practiced type of European massage in the United States. It uses long gliding strokes, kneading, and friction techniques on superficial muscles. Movement travels in the direction of blood flow toward your heart stimulating your circulation through the soft tissues of your body. Oil is used to facilitate the stroking and kneading of your body. This stimulates your circulation.

WESTERN MASSAGE uses methods based on your anatomy and physiology. Manipulation and mind/body strategies attempt to improve personal growth, emotional release, and balance. Esalen massage is a modern variation that focuses on deeper states of relaxation, beneficial states of consciousness, and general well-being. Esalen is slow, rhythmic, and hypnotic and focuses on mind/body integration.

NEUROMUSCULAR MASSAGE applies concentrated finger pressure specifically to your individual muscles. This increases blood flow and releases trigger points. Knots of muscle tension that refer pain to other parts of your body are released with this type of massage. Neuromuscular massage helps to break the cycle of muscle spasm and pain.

DEEP TISSUE MASSAGE uses slow strokes, direct pressure, and friction to release chronic muscle pain. The movements sweep across the grain of your muscles. The practitioner uses his or her fingers, thumbs, or elbows to massage deep within the tissue. This technique is more specific to certain muscles. For example, if you had a sore shoulder, your masseuse or masseur would focus on all layers of your trapezius to get to the root of the problem. Deep tissue massage relaxes your sore muscles.

SPORTS MASSAGE is similar to Swedish and deep tissue but more specific to deal with your sports needs. Sports massage is used before or after your particular event as part of your training and performance. The purpose of sports massage is to promote healing from injuries.

structural functional integration techniques are other mind/body methods of manipulation. Their purpose is to correct inappropriate movement patterns and use manipulation and massage to enhance your muscle tissue. Balance between the nervous system and muscular system is the goal of these programs. These techniques include Rolfing, Hellerwork, the Rosen Method, the Trager Method, the Feldenkrais Method, the Alexander Technique, and Ortho-Bionomy.

- Rolfing attempts to reorder your body by bringing your head, shoulders, thorax, pelvis, and legs into perfect alignment. Rolfing releases adhesions in your muscle fascia. Fascia is the substance that surrounds your muscles. Your fascia is supposed to be supple and flexible. Injury and chronic stress can create sticking points or adhesions, causing your facia to get stuck. Rolfing helps to release this problem.
- Hellerwork teaches you how to stand, sit, walk, and bend appropriately.

- The Rosen Method incorporates touch therapy with a form of psychotherapy. The purpose of Rosen is to release tension and unexpressed feelings.
- The Trager Method teaches you to move freely and relaxed. Your relaxed body helps to focus your mind.
- The Feldenkrais Method improves your flexibility and posture, thereby alleviating muscular tension and pain.
- The Alexander Technique teaches both hands-on and verbal techniques to experience new ways of moving and experiencing.
- Ortho-Bionomyis a process that uses gentle, relaxing movements and postures to help release muscular tension.

ASIAN TECHNIQUES focus on aiding the flow of energy (*qi*) through your body's meridians. Pressure is applied by finger or thumb tips to predetermined points rather than by the sweeping broad strokes as in Western style massage. There are over a dozen varieties of Asian massage and bodywork therapies, but the most common forms in this country are acupressure and shiatsu.

Acupressure and shiatsu are similar techniques of finger pressure massage. They both apply pressure to a pattern of specific points that correspond to the acupuncture points of the body. Pressure is applied with the thumb, finger, and palm. The goal is to balance *qi* flow through the meridians of your body. Muscle tension impairs the flow of *qi*; therefore, the more relaxed you are the better your *qi* can flow. Acupressure is the generic term for this method while shiatsu is the Japanese version.

These Asian methods all make use of energy. There are also other energy programs that are not Asian-based.

THERAPEUTIC TOUCH is based on the idea that the human energy field extends beyond the skin. The practitioner uses his or her hands as sensors to locate problems in your body. Disease is seen as an energy imbalance or blocked energy flow. Assessment is done by passing hands over your body from head to toe at about two to four inches above the surface. With this procedure there is no physical contact made, so these techniques are possible with post surgical patients and burn victims. Therapeutic touch is taught in over eighty universities and thirty countries and is practiced by twenty to thirty thousand health care professionals in the United States and around the world.

REIKI is the Japanese word for universal life force energy. During this procedure the Reiki practitioner serves as a conduit for healing energy coming from the universe. The Reiki energy enters the practitioner through the top of the head and exits through the hands, being directed into your body or energy field. Reiki may be done through clothing and without any physical contact.

REFLEXOLOGY involves the manual stimulation of reflex points on your ears, hands, and feet. Thumb pressure is applied to points that correspond to specific organs of your body. Theoretically, the pressure on these reflex points relieve stress and tension, improving blood supply, unblocking nerve impulses, and helping to restore balance in your body.

ZERO BALANCING is a hands-on method of aligning your body energy with your body structure. The practitioner uses gentle pressure at key areas of your skeleton in order to balance your energy body with your structural body. It is believed that you have an unseen energy glove that surrounds your body. Balancing refers to balancing your energy with your bodily structure.

Massage does improve your circulation and aids in reducing tension. Massage therapy ranges in price from $30 to $60 an hour and is less expensive in rural areas. The cost of specialized techniques are, however, higher. Rolfing, for example, averages about $80 for a ninety-minute session and is usually accomplished in a ten-session series spaced a week apart.

The most common titles for massage therapists are as follows: *Nationally Certified in Therapeutic Massage and Bodywork*. This title designates the person has completed the requirements for and passed the National Certification Board for Therapeutic Massage and Bodywork (N.C.B.T.M.B.). This is the leading national certification exam.

Massage Practitioner (M.P.). This title is often used by practitioners whose training is less extensive than that required for certification by schools or by the AMTA as a massage therapist.

Certified Massage Therapist (C.M.T.). This is a voluntary, professional, non-governmental certification from organizations that can attest to the therapist's competency. This is granted by many massage therapy schools, which may or may not meet AMTA standards for training. Thus the quality of this credential depends on the quality of the certifier and its standards. (For example, even a person who has only taken an eight-hour course can claim to be certified.)

Registered Massage Therapist (R.M.T.). This is a form of voluntary licensing for the use of a specific professional title. Rarely used in the United States, some Canadian provinces use this to designate government licensing. At one time it also designated a special credential for members of the AMTA who had advanced training in therapeutic massage and passed a special exam, but this usage has been discontinued.

Licensed Massage Therapist (L.M.T.). This refers to occupational licensing by a state or local government. Nineteen states have licensing laws requiring massage therapists to meet minimum standards of training. The basic requirement is usually five hundred hours of classroom training with instructors present, followed by a written and practical exam.

The American Massage Therapy Association is the predominant organization for massage therapists with over eighteen thousand members, representing all fifty states, D.C., the Virgin Islands, and several foreign countries.

Modeling Your Inner Force

Awareness of your surroundings can help you achieve your mind/body goals. You can use nature as role model to enhance your mindfulness. The natural inner force inherent in each species of animals is a role model for advanced training. For example, the inner force of the cobra inspires speed and quickness. You can summon the single-minded tenacity of the tiger during combat or model the inner force of the lion: feel proud and unbeatable walk with confidence, strength, and majesty.

The following are tips that will help you develop your inner force.

INNER FORCE STRATEGIES

1. Develop a crystal clear visual picture of your inner force.

2. Re-create the attitude and feelings of your inner force.

3. Possess the cat-quick, agile, fast-stepping power of your inner force.

4. Integrate your inner force with your physical movement so that each attack and defense comes from within.

5. Become one with your inner force.

6. In spare moments, imagine and visualize the power of your inner force.

7. Practice inner force movements in real life.

Over 500 students taking a variety of required physical education classes at the Northeast Texas Community College were administered a pre-test assessing their focus, sense of purpose, feelings, motivation, work and play, breathing, psychological stress, relaxation, leisure time, and overall well-being. Results demonstrated many students have goals but find it difficult to go from ambition to action. Most, however, had a purpose and were motivated. They were in touch with their feelings and focused. Many enjoyed their chosen field and felt good about themselves. However, all reported being under a great deal of stress and not able to use their leisure time effectively. Rarely did they take part in relaxation or recreation.

Take this time to evaluate yourself and be objective. Answer the questions below as honestly as you can. Review you answers and reflect. Be mindful and adjust whatever it is in your life that you are not comfortable with.

ANSWER TRUE OR FALSE TO THE LEFT OF EACH QUESTION

PURPOSE

____ I believe my life to have direction and meaning.

____ My life is exciting and challenging.

____ I have goals in my life.

____ I am achieving my goals.

____ I look forward to the future as an opportunity for further growth.

____ My daily life is a source of pleasure to me.

MOTIVATION

_____ I am not easily discouraged.

_____ I rarely let myself down.

_____ I set goals regularly.

_____ I keep promises to myself.

_____ I have structure in my life.

_____ I have a relaxed lifestyle.

_____ If I could do things over again, I would not change much.

_____ I have reached many of my goals in life.

_____ I am not disappointed with any area of my life.

_____ I am happy.

RELAXATION AND LEISURE

_____ I have a supportive family.

_____ I actively spend time with a hobby.

_____ I participate in social activities regularly.

_____ I am close to my ideal body weight.

_____ I practice relaxation techniques such as meditation or prayer regularly.

_____ I exercise at least thirty minutes three times per week.

_____ I eat balanced meals throughout the day.

_____ I do something "just for myself" regularly.

_____ I have a favorite "relaxation place" in my home.

_____ I am good at staying on my schedule.

_____ I do strength training at least two times each week.

_____ I use part of my leisure time to do activities with my family.

_____ It is easy for me to relax and express my feelings.

_____ I prepare for events or activities so I am not required to rush around at the last minute.

_____ I can talk to family and friends about personal problems.

_____ I sleep about eight hours each night.

_____ I do not have trouble falling asleep at night.

____ I do not have too much trouble waking in the morning.

____ I do not awaken during the night.

____ When I awaken in the morning I am energized and ready to go.

____ I am energized throughout the day.

BREATHING

____ I stop during the day to become aware of the way I am breathing.

____ I meditate, pray, or relax at least fifteen minutes each day.

____ I enjoy work and do not find it overly stressful.

____ My personal relationships are satisfying.

____ I take time out for deep breathing several times a day.

____ I have plenty of energy.

____ I am at peace with myself.

WORK AND PLAY

____ I regularly try to be creative.

____ I enjoy spending time without structured activities and make an effort to do so.

____ I change my work into play.

____ At times I allow myself to do nothing.

____ My work is rewarding.

____ I am proud of my accomplishments.

____ I am playful and friends support my playfulness.

____ I have one activity (hobby, sport, etc.) I enjoy regularly.

FOCUS

____ It is easy for me to concentrate.

____ I am conscious of changes (such as breathing pattern, muscle tension, skin moisture, etc.) in my body in response to certain thoughts.

____ I notice my perceptions of the world are colored by my thoughts.

____ I am aware that my thoughts are influenced by my environment.

142

_____ Rather than worry about a problem when I can do nothing about it, I temporarily shelve it and get on with important matters.

_____ I use my creativity in many aspects of my life.

FEELING

_____ I am able to say "no" to people without feeling guilty.

_____ I laugh often and easily.

_____ I have at least five close friends.

_____ I like myself and look forward to the rest of my life.

_____ I easily express concern, love, and warmth to those I care about.

_____ I can ask for help when needed.

MANIPULATION CHECK

_____ Am I energized?

_____ Am I calm?

_____ Am I confident?

_____ Am I happy?

_____ Am I relaxed?

_____ Am I focused?

_____ Am I motivated?

_____ Am I balanced?

_____ Am I secure?

_____ Am I hopeful?

_____ Am I growing?

_____ Am I satisfied?

ASPIRATION

- Goal setting is the aim or purpose of an action.
- Identify what you are attempting to achieve.

- Goal setting improves performance. It provides direction and guides you on your journey.
- Goals direct your attention toward accomplishing the task.
- Identify your goals.
- Set short- and long-term goals.
- Set performance goals instead of outcome goals.

Some of us have an inner drive to succeed. It appears inborn. Perhaps a turn of events or a single circumstance was responsible. After further observation we see that there was no magic moment. We are not born with mental skills. They must be learned and practiced. The ability to concentrate, to relax under pressure, and to maintain your confidence are not magically achieved. Successful are those who can control their thoughts and emotions on a consistent basis and can maintain a high level of excellence from day to day. The fate of you success lies in your hands, and your hands alone. Go for it.

Resources

Academy for Guided Imagery provides training for professionals in the use of guided imagery. Address: P.O. Box 2070, Mill Valley, CA 94942, phone (800) 726-2070 or (415) 389-9324, FAX (415) 389-9342.

American Academy of Reflexology conducts training in ear, hand, and foot reflexology and can provide referrals to certified practitioners. Address: 606 E. Magnolia Blvd., Suite B. Burbank, CA 91501, phone (818) 841-7741.

American Chronic Pain Association manages a list of over five hundred support groups internationally, and publishes workbooks and a newsletter. Address: P.O. Box 850, Rocklin, CA 95677, phone (916) 632-0922.

American Council of Hypnotist Examiners (ACHE) provides a referral list of professionally trained hypnotists and hypnotherapists certified by ACHE. It does not require licenser in a health or mental health profession. Address: 312 Riverdale Dr., Glendale, CA 91204, phone (818) 242-5378.

American Society of Clinical Hypnosis (ASCH) is the largest and most highly accredited organization for hypnotherapists. The ASCH sponsors the American Board of Clinical Hypnosis, which certifies practitioners, and maintains a referral list of professionally trained and licensed hypnotherapists. Address: 2200 East Devon Ave., Suite 291, Des Plaines, IL 60018, phone (708) 297-3317, FAX (708) 297-7309.

Associated Bodywork and Massage Professionals (ABMP) provides professional support and legislative advocacy for massage therapists and bodyworkers. Membership is of two levels: practitioner level requires one hundred hours of training. Professional level requires five hundred hours or state licenser or registration. ABMP also publishes *Massage and Bodywork Quarterly*. Address: 28677 Buffalo Park Rd., Evergreen CO 80439, phone (303) 674-8478.

Biofeedback Certification Institute of America provides a directory of certified biofeedback practitioners, including their background and experience. Address: 10200 W.44th Ave., Suite 304, Wheatridge, CO 80033, phone (303) 420-2902.

Center for Attitudinal Healing has support groups throughout the nation for people with chronic or life threatening illness. Address: 33 Buchanan, Sausalito, CA 94965, phone (415) 331-6161.

Center for Mind/Body Medicine has both residential and outpatient programs. Developed under the guidance of Deepak Chopra, M.D., it also provides education and training programs in Ayurveda for laypeople and health care providers. Address: P.O. Box 1048, La Jolla, CA 92038, phone (619) 794-2425, FAX (619) 794-2440.

Feldenkrais Guild. Only people trained by Moshe Feldenkrais or graduates of guild accredited training programs are eligible to be members of the guild. Practitioner members are qualified teachers of Awareness Through Movement and Functional Integration. Associate members are qualified teachers of Awareness Through Movement. The professional training program spans 160 days over three and a half years. The guild publishes a directory of certified practitioners. Address: 706 Ellsworth St., P.O. Box 489, Albany, OR 97321-0143, phone (800) 775-2118 or (503) 926-0981.

Hellerwork, Inc. Training is a 1,250-hour program leading to certification as a Hellerwork practitioner. Training is offered internationally. Address: 406 Berry St., Mt. Shasta, CA 96067, phone (800) 392-3900 or (916) 926-2500.

Insight Meditation Society and *Insight Meditation West* offer workshops and retreats nationwide in mindfulness meditation, also called vipassana meditation. Address: IMS, Pleasant St., Bare, MA 01005, phone (508) 355-4378; IMW, P.O. Box 909, Woodier, CA 94973, phone (415) 488-0164.

International Institute of Reflexology conducts two-day trainings nationally and internationally and a certification exam in the Ingham Method of reflexology. They also can provide referrals to trained practitioners. Address: 5650 First Avenue North, P.O. Box 12642, St. Petersburg, FL 33733, phone (813) 343-4811.

Maharishi Ayur-Ved Products International provides referrals to local resources for training in transcendental meditation (TM). Address: P.O. Box 49667, Colorado Springs, CO 80949-9667, phone (800) 255-8332.

MindBody Medical Institute, Division of Behavioral Medicine, New England Deaconess Hospital offers group mind/body programs for different illnesses. They also have affiliate programs nationwide and conduct clinical training several times each year under the direction of Herbert Benson, M.D., and faculty. Address: 1 Deaconess Rd., Boston, MA 02215, phone (617) 632-9525, FAX (617) 632-7383.

Morris, P. L., R. G. Robinson, P. Andrzejewski, J. Samuels, and T. R. Price. 1993. Association of depression with ten-year poststroke mortality. *American Journal of Psychiatry* 150:124-29.

North American Society of Teachers of the Alexander Technique (NASTAT) formed in 1987 to educate the public about the Alexander Technique, to establish and maintain standards for certification of teachers and teacher training courses in the United States, and to ensure that the educational principles of the Alexander Technique are upheld. It publishes a directory of certified teachers. Training to become a teacher takes three years (sixteen hundred hours). Address: P.O. Box 112484, Tacoma, WA 98411-2484, phone (800) 473-0620 or (206) 627-3766.

Nurse Healers Professional Associates, Inc., provides information about Therapeutic Touch and training for health care providers. The length of trainings varies and there is no formal certification. Address: P.O. Box 444, Allison Park, PA 15101, phone (412) 355-8476.

Rolf Institute of Structural Integration. The training is typically twelve months long for basic certification. A Certified Advanced Rolfer is one who has practiced at least five years and has taken an additional six weeks training. A list of certified practitioners is available. Address: 205 Canyon Blvd., Boulder, CO 80302, phone (800) 530-8875.

Rosen Method Professional Association. Certification training is two years plus an eighteen-month internship. Certified practitioners must also hold a state-approved massage certificate. A directory of practitioners is available from the association. Address: 2550 Shattuck Ave., Box 49, Berkeley, CA 94704, phone (510) 644-4166.

Stress Reduction Clinic, University of Massachusetts Medical Center, directed by Jon Kabat-Zinn, Ph.D., conducts an eight week program and a five-day residential program in mindfulness training and stress reduction. Address: UMMC, Worcester, MA 01655, phone (508) 856-1616.

Trager Institute. Training for Trager practitioners takes a minimum of 269 hours usually over at least six months. A list of certified practitioners is available. Address: 33 Millwood St., Mill Valley, CA 94941, phone (415) 388-2688, FAX (415) 388-2710.

Wellness Community has chapters throughout the nation that conduct support groups for people with chronic or life threatening illness. Address: 2716 Ocean Park Blvd., Suite 1040, Santa Monica, CA 90405, phone (310)314-2555

Zero Balancing Association offers training in this method, a fifty-hour basic course, and an eighteen-month certification program. Address: P.O. Box 1727, Capitola, CA 95010, phone (408) 476-0665

References

Benson, H., J. Beary, and M. Carol. 1974. The relaxation response. *Psychiatry* 37:37-46.

Benson, H.1977. Systemic hypertension and the relaxation response. *The New England Journal of Medicine* 296:1152-56.

Byers, D. 1991. *Better Health with Foot Reflexalogy.* St. Petersburg, FL: Ingham Publishing, Inc.

Collinge, W.1988. Psychosocial outcomes of complementary cancer therapy. *Proceedings of the Society of Behavioral Medicine, Ninth Annual Scientific Sessions.* Boston: 60-61.

Dossey, L. 1989. Mind Beyond Body, in *Healers on Healing,* edited by R. Carlson and B. Shield. Los Angeles: Jeremy P. Tarcher, Inc.: 174.

Fakouri, C., and T. Jones. Relaxation Rx: slow stroke back rub. 1987. *Journal of Gerontological Nursing* 13(2):32-35.

Field, T., C. Morrow, C. Valdeon, et al. 1992. Massage reduces anxiety in child and adolescent psychiatric patients. *Journal of the American Academy of Child and Adolescent Psychiatry* 31(1):125-31.

Field, T., S. Schanberg, F. Scafidi, et al. 1986. Tactile/kinesthetic stimulation effects on preterm neonates. *Pediatrics* (May) 77(5):654-158.

Glaser, R., J. Rice, C. Speicher, et al. 1985. Stress-related impairments in cellular immunity. *Psychiatry Research* 16:233-39.

Glaser, R., J. Rice, C. Speicher, J. Stout, and J. Kiecolt-Glaser. 1986. Stress depresses interferon production concomitant with a decrease in natural killer cell activity. *Behavioral Neuroscience* 100(5):675-78.

Gruber, B., and N. Hall.1988. Immune system and psychological changes in metastatic cancer patients using relaxation and guided imagery: a pilot study. Scandinavian *Journal of Behavior Therapy* 17:25-45.

Hunt, V. V., W. W. Massey, R. Weinberg, R. Bruyere, and P. M. Hahn. 1977. *A study of structural integration from neuromuscular, energy field, and emotional approaches.* Boulder, CO: Rolf Institute of Structural Integration.

Kiecolt-Glaser, J., W. Garner, C. Speicher, G. Penn, J. Holliday, and R. Glaser. 1984. Psychosocial modifiers of immunocompetence in medical students. *Psychosomatic Medicine* 46:7-14.

Oleson, T., and W. Flocco. 1993. Randomized controlled study of premenstrual symptoms treated with ear, hand, and foot reflexology. *Obstetrics and Gynecology* (December) 82(6):906-110.

Olness, K. 1993. Hypnosis: the power of attention. in *Mind/body medicine: How to use your mind for better health,* edited by D. Goleman and J. Gurin. Yonkers, NY: Consumer Reports Books: 278.

Ornish, D., S. E. Brown, L. W. Scherwitz, J. H. Billings, W. T. Armstrong, T. A. Ports, 15.

Orme-Johnson, D. 1987. Medical care utilization and the transcendental meditation program. *Psychosomatic Medicine* 49:493-507.

Weintraub, M. 1992. Shiatsu, Swedish muscle massage, and trigger point suppression in spinal pain syndrome. Massage Therapy Journal (Summer) 31 (3):99-109. Also published in *American Journal of Pain Management* (April 1992) 2(2):74-78.

Wells, J., G. Howard, W. Nowlin, and M. Vargas. 1986. Presurgical anxiety and post-surgical pain and adjustment: effects of stress inoculation procedure. *Journal of Consulting and Clinical Psychology* 57:831-53.

Yoachim, G. 1983. The effects of two stress management techniques on feelings of well-being in patients with inflammatory bowel disease. *Nursing Papers* 15(47):5-18.

Glossary

Acetylcholine: A neurotransmitter that slows your heart rate. It is controlled by your parasympathetic nervous system (PNS).

Active Recovery: Toxins accumulate in your muscles after exercise. These waste products are drastically reduced if you perform some type of activity after your workout. Walking, pedaling, or light jogging for ten to fifteen minutes will greatly improve the breakdown of metabolites to reduce unwanted stiffness and soreness.

Acupuncture: A way to contact the electrical centers of your body and influence the flow of energy. Its purpose is to bring about a balance between positive and negative (yin-yang) forces. The qi energy travels through your body by means of pathways called meridians. Needles stimulate various points along these meridians.

Adipose Tissue: a.k.a. fat. This is a yellowish substance within your fat cells.

Aerobic Exercise: Aerobic means with oxygen. Aerobic exercise is the exercise during which the energy needed is supplied by the oxygen inspired. Move your large muscle groups in a rhythmic fashion and you are doing aerobics. Walking, jogging, stairclimbing, swimming, and jumping rope are examples.

Aldosterone: Your adrenal gland secretes this hormone. It functions in regulation of sodium, chloride, and potassium.

Alexander Method: The Alexander Method is a set of techniques for unlearning old bad habits so your natural body can take over.

Alimentary Canal: Another word for your gastrointestinal (GI) tract.

Allergies: Allergies occur when your immune system reacts to pollen, mold, or dust. Your body perceives these irritants as if they were alien invaders. Your symptoms include: watery nasal discharge; sneezing; coughing; itchy eyes, nose, and throat; nasal congestion; and dark circles under your eyes.

Alpha State: A brain wave pattern characterized by relaxed-concentration.

Amygdala: This is the part of your brain that is involved with emotion and memory.

Anaerobic Exercise: Anaerobic means without oxygen. Anaerobic exercise is the exercise during which the energy needed is provided without the utilization of inspired oxygen. High intensity, short duration activities are anaerobic. Weight training, sprinting, basketball, racketball, and tennis are anaerobic.

Androgens: These are your male steroid hormones. They are produced in your adrenal glands and ovaries in women. These are the types of steroids that help you to build muscle.

Anemia: Your body uses iron to make red blood cells. If your iron levels drop, then your body loses its ability to manufacture red blood cells. The fewer red blood cells you have, the less hemoglobin. As your hemoglobin drops, the ability of your blood to carry oxygen decreases and you have less energy. Symptoms of anemia include fatigue, shortness of breath, dizziness, light-headedness, fainting, and decreased resistance to colds and other infections.

Aphasia: Difficulty speaking or understanding language. It usually occurs after a stroke. Aphasia affects the left hemisphere of the brain, where language is processed.

Applied Kiniesiology: a structure used to analyze your structural, chemical, and mental aspects of health. Muscle testing, postural analysis, and gait analysis are used to treat functional problems. Applied kinesiologists use joint manipulations, myofacial therapies, cranial techniques, meridian therapy, clinical nutrition, and dietary management.

Arousal: a.k.a. activation level.

Arrhythmia: An abnormal heart rhythm. This is usually caused by a problem with your heart's electrical system.

Arteriosclerosis: a.k.a. hardening of the arteries It refers to the fact that your arteries may become hard and brittle through the deposition of calcium on artery walls.

Artery: A type of blood vessel that carries blood away from your heart.

Association: Focusing on the activity you are performing.

Asthma: The wheeze of asthma is caused by contraction of the muscular walls of the small breathing tubes in your lungs. The narrowed air tube creates a turbulent air flow. This causes the wheezing or whistling when you breathe. Because the tubes into the lung are narrowed, less air can get in and this decreases the oxygen supply to your body. The pathological muscular contraction of your breathing tubes can be stimulated by a wide range of substances such as inhaled dust or pollen, and various foods.

Atkins Diet: A high protein, low carbohydrate, high fat diet that has not been shown to be beneficial to long term weight loss.

Atrial Fibrillation: A heart rhythm problem where your atria quivers ineffectually. This allows blood to sit idly, and nonproductively, in your left atrium.

Audience Arousal: When someone is watching you perform a task, it increases your arousal.

Autonomic Nervous System (ANS): This is the part of your nervous system that controls involuntary, automatic, process. Examples include your heart beat and breathing.

Axon: A part of the neuron that transmits a signal to a cell.

Basal Metabolic Rate (BMR): Your BMR is the amount of calories your body burns at rest. Your BMR includes sixty percent of your caloric burn from your functioning organs. Twenty-five percent from your muscles, ten percent from your bones, and 5 percent from fat.

Bioenergetics: According to this theory, your body expresses everything that happens to you. Bioenergetic exercises are designed to open blocked or tensed areas of your body. As your body relaxes, so do your emotions and attitudes.

Biofeedback: Technological devices monitor unconscious processes and feedback this information to your conscious mind. This way, your conscious mind learns to control your unconscious.

Biorhythms: This theory suggests your physical, mental, and emotional cycles all have special relationships to each other. By charting your physical, creative, intellectual, and emotional cycles, you can learn to take advantage of these systems to enhance your life.

Brain Stem: This is the part of your brain that controls your breathing, heart rate, and other vital functions.

Breathing During Exercise: You could virtually hold your breath while lifting weights, sprinting to your mailbox, or serving a tennis ball. But don't try it. Exhale with exertion and you will perform better, without blowing a gasket.

Burn Fat: You burn fat all day and all night long. To burn fat most efficiently, a comfortable but challenging pace is your best steady-state speed to burn fat.

Calorie: Some consider calories the enemy. Fat calories, in particular. You can get fat on too many fat, protein, or carbohydrate calories. Your body needs calories for growth, repair, and energy.

Cardiac Output: The amount of blood that your heart can pump in one minute.

Cerebellum: This is the part of your brain that coordinates your movements.

Cerebral Cortex: This is the part of your brain that is involved in thought, language, and memory.

Chiropractic: The study of health and disease from a structural point of view. Special consideration is given to your spine and nerves. A practitioner who treats disease by manipulation of the spine and other body structures.

Controllability: Your ability to control the mental picture you have created in an attempt to improve your performance.

Dissociation: Keeping your mind on something else, rather than thinking about the activity you are doing.

Dopamine: This is a neurotransmitter that helps you to move comfortably and smoothly.

Epinephrine: a.k.a. adrenaline it is a chemical that can act as a neurotransmitter or a hormone. It constricts your blood vessels and increases your heart rate.

Exercise stress test: A test used to determine your heart's response to exercise.

Fat Cells: You developed your fat cells during the third trimester in your mother's womb (so blame it on your mom), your first year of life (that's her fault again), and during puberty. It is also theorized you can add fat cells during pregnancy, and during explosive weight gain in adulthood.

Fat Loss: You cannot lose fat cells, unless you undergo liposuction. You may however, decrease the fat within each of your cells with proper diet and exercise.

Fatty acids: These are the primary building blocks of fats (lipids).

Fine Motor Task: A small muscle movement such as putting in golf.

Flow: A mindful experience where there is no ego, competition, anxiety, or boredom. Flow is an alpha state that allows you to perform your activity on automatic.

Frequency: How many times a week you work out.

Glucose: The body's main source of energy. Glucose is a sugar that comes mainly from the digestion of carbohydrates.

Gross Motor Task: A large muscle movement such as pushing a refrigerator.

Heart Rate Training: Monitoring your heart rate while you perform anaerobic and aerobic training to reach certain heart rate levels.

Histamine: A chemical present in specific cells throughout your body. It is a mediator of allergic reactions.

Hormones: These are chemical released from glands into your bloodstream. They affect organs or tissues elsewhere in your body.

Hypertension: a.k.a. high blood pressure. High blood pressure is a major risk factor for stroke. Hypertension causes excess stress on the walls of your blood vessels and damages their delicate inner lining.

Hypertrophy: a.k.a. muscle growth.

Imagery: A psychological strategy designed to help you improve your physical performance.

Inflammation: Inflammation is a process that occurs in response to a range of traumas from sunburn and wounds, to infection and auto-immune conditions. Whatever the cause, the process leads to warmth, redness, swelling, and pain.

Insomnia: Insomnia, or sleeplessness may be caused by a variety of triggers. The key to successful treatment of insomnia is to find the cause and deal with it. Whether the cause is emotional, physical, or environmental (a snoring spouse), seek out the cause of your insomnia to uncover the cure.

Instructor Motivation: A group exercise leader can increase your motivation to burn an additional two calories per minute.

Insulin: A hormone produced by your pancreas. Insulin helps blood glucose (sugar) get into your cells.

Intensity: How hard you work out.

Internal Obliques: Your internal obliques are beneath your external obliques. They form the shape of a roof top. Your right internal oblique turns you to the right and your left internal oblique turns you to the left.

Limbic System: The part of your brain that contains your amygdala, hippocampus, and the basal ganglia. It affects emotion, memory, and certain aspects of movement.

Lipase: An enzyme that is secreted by your pancreas that helps digest fats.

Lipids: a.k.a. Fats, oils, and waxes. They serve as building blocks for cells or as energy sources for the body.

Lipoproteins: These are protein covered fat particles. They enable cholesterol and triglycerides to move easily through your blood.

Massage: Muscles typically tighten after exercise. The speed of recovery is directly related to the amount of blood that can enter the muscle to provide the necessary food and oxygen. Deep massage immediately after exercise encourages blood to enter a more relaxed muscle. Get a massage fifteen minutes after exercising, and several times during the rest of the day. Each session only needs to be 45–60 seconds.

Mind/Body Recovery: Successful rehabilitation begins with learning about your injury. Know the extent of your injury, what your recovery time will be, and what you must do to recover. A recent cool study showed that just by thinking about doing a biceps curl, you actually produce muscular activity in your biceps.

Minerals: Some athletes think they need doses of minerals to enhance their physical training. But studies show that, except for iron (particularly among female athletes), the mineral needs of highly trained athletes are similar to those of the general population. Furthermore, physical training does not inordinately deplete minerals.

Monounsaturated fats (MUFAs): a.k.a. the good fats. Ufatty acids, abundant in olive, peanut, sesame, and canola oils, in which one pair of hydrogen atoms in each molecule has been replaced by a double bond.

Motility: This refers to the speed and capability of your digestive tract to propel its contents through your system.

Movement Time: From the moment you begin your movement, until you complete it.

Muscle Cramp: A muscle cramp is when your muscle contracts and shortens causing a sudden, severe pain. Muscle cramps are mostly caused by overexertion and dehydration. When you dehydrated, there is an electrolyte imbalance and your muscles to cramp up. Electrolytes are minerals such as sodium, magnesium, calcium and potassium. An imbalance occurs when we have too much or too little of one or more electrolytes in our system. The main electrolytes affecting muscle cramping are potassium, sodium, and calcium.

Muscle Metabolism: You should eat enough calories to maintain your BMR. If not, your metabolism will slow, and you will store fat more efficiently.

Muscle/Fat: Muscle does not turn into fat. Muscle and fat are two separate entities. If you lose muscle your metabolism slows. If you eat more calories than you burn, you gain fat.

Muscle: Seventy-five percent of your muscle is water, twenty percent is protein, and five percent minerals. You have more than 400 voluntary muscles in your body. Muscle makes up about half of your body weight. The more muscle you have the more calories your body burns. Muscle is metabolically active.

Myofascial Release: Myofascial release is using pressure from your arms and fingers to lengthen muscle and connective tissue. It is used in combination with physical therapy methods to relieve pain and stiffness.

Neuron: A nerve cell.

Norepinephrine: This neurotransmitter constricts your blood vessels. It is released by your sympathetic nervous system.

Optimum Level of Arousal: A sate of being not too bored or too anxious. At a perfect energy level for the activity you are performing.

Overtraining: The same motivation that you have to train hard and perform well can get you into trouble.

Parasympathetic Nervous System (PNS): One of the two branches of your autonomic nervous system. It helps to regulate digestion, circulation, voiding, and other bodily functions.

Parathyroid Hormone: A hormone, made by four tiny pieces of tissue near your thyroid. It prevents your level of blood calcium from going to low.

Passive Stretching: Using a partner to take one of your limbs through a range of motion.

Peripheral Vision: Side vision. This is what you can see outside of your direct line of vision.

Pilates: Pilates(puh-la-tease) is named after Joseph Pilates who developed it in Germany in the 1920s. It was a favorite exercise for dancers who wanted to strengthen their muscles and soothe their aches and strains. Now it's the rage among those burned out on regular weight training. Proponents of Pilates suggest that it lengthens and strengthens muscle, while improving balance and posture.

Placebo Effect: a.k.a. sugar pill, it is an inactive substance given to satisfy a patients demand for medicine. From chromium picolinate to shark cartilage, people think more of supplements than they are worth. Folks swear to me the benefits of colloidal minerals and magnets. Benjamin Franklin painted blocks of wood black. People thought they were magnets. They slept with these blocks of wood because they believed magnets cured arthritis. Miraculously, they were healed. The blocks of wood worked!

Polyunsaturated fats (PUFAs): a.k.a. the good fats. These are fatty acids found in soybean, corn, cottonseed, safflower, and sunflower oils. Two or more pairs of hydrogen atoms in each molecule have been replaced by double bonds.

Proprioceptive Neuromuscular Facilitation (PNF): A type of stretching where you take your partners limb through a passive stretch. When your partner feels tension in the muscle, he/she presses against you for three seconds. Then he/she relaxes and you once again attempt to move your partners limb a little deeper into the stretch. The purpose of PNF is to activate your golgi tendon organ to relax your muscle and provide for a further stretch.

Proprioceptive Training: a.k.a. balance training.

Pseudoephedrine: A decongestant drug.

Pursed Lipped Breathing: Used to slow your exhalation by forming your lips as if you were whistling.

Reaction time: From the moment you think about starting your movement, until your muscles take action.

Reiki: Reiki is a hands on, non-invasive healing technique. A form of like a Japanese form of acupressure. The client participates in their own healing. The reiki practitioner is a channel and a clear vessel through which the healing energy flows. Reiki energy allows us to heal ourselves spiritually, emotionally, mentally, and physically.

Relaxed Concentration: An alpha brain wave pattern where your mind and body are relaxed, but you are exquisitely focused on your task at hand.

Rolfing: Rolfing involves movement education and body restructuring. It relieves tension and helps to align your body parts in perfect posture. Since you are balanced, you spend less effort fighting gravity. The massage technique called rolfing was designed to fight the effects of gravity. Some folks with back and neck problems say it releases their tension and relieves their pain.

Saturated fats: a.k.a. bad fats. These are fatty acids, abundant in red meat, lard, butter, hard cheeses, and some vegetable oils (palm, coconut, and cocoa butter) and partially hydrogenated oils. Each molecule carries the maximum amount of hydrogen atoms.

Shiatsu: A Japanese form of acupuncture. Finger pressure is applied to acupuncture meridian points by a practitioner. The pressure stimulates and balances the energy flowing through your body.

Spinning: Group indoor stationary cycling.

Starting a Program: Your body burns more calories sprinting than walking for the same time period. But begin easy. When you become more fit you can workout harder.

Static Stretching: Holding your stretch at a point of tension.

Stepper Machines: The speed that you step does not affect your caloric burn because the slower you go, the deeper you step.

Strain: Damage to a muscle or tendon.

Stress: Stress is the response of your body to any demand. Just staying alive creates demands on your body, so you are always under stress. Even while you sleep, your body continues to function. Stress cannot be avoided nor should it be. Stress is linked to problems like high blood pressure and heart disease. It also exacerbates headaches, backaches, and digestive troubles. Stress can make your body aches more painful, your queasy stomach more upset, or worsen any of your symptoms, no matter what the original cause.

Stretch Reflex: When you stretch a muscle too hard or too fast, it will contract to protect itself.

Stretching: A combination of massage and stretching is the perfect medicine for tightened muscles after a workout. Use massage to relax your muscles. Now your muscle is prepared for recovery stretching. This keeps your muscles from tightening and shortens recovery time.

Substrate Cycling: Athletes adjust their voluminous training to their eating so that they can eat voraciously to make up for caloric loss, and workout again and eat, and workout

Supine: a.k.a. lying on your back.

Supplements: If you are going to use supplements, they should be used in addition to an eating and exercise program, not in replacement of. As long as supplement companies claims their products are foods, their advertising is virtually unregulated. Be careful.

Sympathetic Nervous System (SNS): One of two divisions of your autonomic nervous system. Your SNS prepares your body for action. Your blood pressure, heart and breathing rate increase to prepare for an emergency.

Synapse: A tiny space between an axon terminal that fires off a chemical signal and the neuron that receives it.

Taijiquan (Tai Chi Chuan): A Chinese martial art form of movement meditation, combining concentration, coordinated breathing, and a series of slow, graceful body movements. Taiji is practiced as a meditation, for health, and as a self-defense.

Testosterone: This is a male hormone. It stimulates bone and muscle growth and sexual development.

Training Motivation: Get a healthy perspective. Make friends with your body. It deserves your kindness. Then, make better choices. Walk away from sedentary life. Include more physical activity and healthier foods into your day. Soon you'll feel better both mentally and physically.

Trigger Point: A painful area to the touch, that when palpated, elicits pain elsewhere in your body. Locate a tender, nodular area within one of your muscles. This is called your trigger point. Gently massage it. Your goal is to restore normal, rich blood and oxygen flow to all parts your muscle. Trigger points strangulate areas of muscles, cutting off the normal nutrition and lifeline, compromising your muscles' function.

Trypsin: An enzyme that is secreted by the pancreas. It helps you to digest proteins.

Vitamins: Vitamins assist chemical reactions in your body. There are thirteen known vitamins: Four are fat-soluble—A, D, E, and K—which your body is able to store in amounts large enough to last for months. There are nine water-soluble vitamins—C (ascorbic acid), and the B-complex vitamins—B1 (thiamin), B2 (riboflavin), B6 (pyridoxine), B12, niacin, folic acid, biotin, and pantothenic acid. Your body needs replenishment of these vitamins regularly.

warmup: Warm up before your martial arts training. Stretch afterwards. A warm up gives your joints a five to ten percent increase in synovial fluid. Stretch after your workout when your muscles are thoroughly heated up.

Yoga: Yoga techniques and postures help your flexibility and mental focus.

Index

ABOUT THE AUTHOR

Tom Seabourne, Ph.D., exercise science, is ACSM, CSCS and ACE certified. Tom is a two-time All-American in Taekwondo and holds several ultra-endurance national cycling records. He finished in the top ten in the Race Across America and was featured as *Sports Illustrated* Athlete of the Month. He is a former collegiate tennis player and two-time National AAU Heavyweight taekwondo Champion, Pan American Champion, and World Silver Medalist. Tom has written over 200 articles and has eight published books on fitness topics including self-defense, mind-body fitness, and cross training. He writes weekly fitness columns for the *Longview News Journal* and is the fitness consultant for www.fitnesslink.com. Tom was the chairman of the 2000 USTU safety committee for the Sydney Olympics and is the Keiser Power Pacing national spokesman. He travels internationally providing workshops on mind/body unity, athletic programming, and exercise analysis. He has been featured nationally on ESPN, Fox and Friends, and *CBS Inside Fitness*. Tom resides in Mt. Pleasant, Texas with his wife and five children.

BOOKS & VIDEOS FROM YMAA